Table of Content

03
Medical Cannabis is Saving Lives

06
Fern

11
Should you Drink Matcha Tea Regularly

18
Lab-Grown Human Skin To Reduce Animal Testing

19
Starting a Plant- Based "Eat To Live" Life

21
The Benefits Of Discovering Transitions Foods, For a Plant-Based Diet

24
Your Whole-Food, Plant-Based Diet— The Foods You'll Love

25
How To Transition To A Plant-Based Diet

31
The Benefits Of A Whole-Food, Plant-Based Diet

34
Healing with hemp: Glow Holistic's Farm

37
The Basic Principles Of Therapy

42
Finding Oneness In Diversity

45
Mindfulness

47
Individuality in Judaism

MAGAZINE TITLE | 2020 ISSUE

Medical Cannabis is Saving Lives

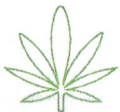

"Medical cannabis laws are associated with significantly lower state-level opioid overdose mortality rates."

In an analysis of death certificate data from 1999 to 2010, we found that states with medical cannabis laws had lower mean opioid analgesic overdose mortality rates compared with states without such laws. This finding persisted when excluding intentional overdose deaths (ie, suicide), suggesting that medical cannabis laws are associated with lower opioid analgesic overdose mortality among individuals using opioid analgesics for medical indications. Similarly, the association between medical cannabis laws and lower opioid analgesic overdose mortality rates persisted when including all deaths related to heroin, even if no opioid analgesic was present, indicating that lower rates of opioid analgesic overdose mortality were not offset by higher rates of heroin overdose mortality. Although the exact mechanism is unclear, our results suggest a link between medical cannabis laws and lower opioid analgesic overdose mortality.

Approximately 60% of all opioid analgesic overdoses occur among patients who have legitimate prescriptions from a single provider. This group may be sensitive to medical cannabis laws; patients with chronic noncancer pain who would have otherwise initiated opioid analgesics may choose medical cannabis instead. Although evidence for the analgesic properties of cannabis is limited, it may provide analgesia for some individuals. In addition, patients already receiving opioid analgesics who start medical cannabis treatment may experience improved analgesia and decrease their opioid dose, thus potentially decreasing their dose-dependent risk of overdose. Finally, if medical cannabis laws lead to decreases in polypharmacy—particularly with benzodiazepines—in people taking opioid analgesics, overdose risk would be decreased. Further analyses examining the association between medical cannabis laws and patterns of opioid analgesic use and

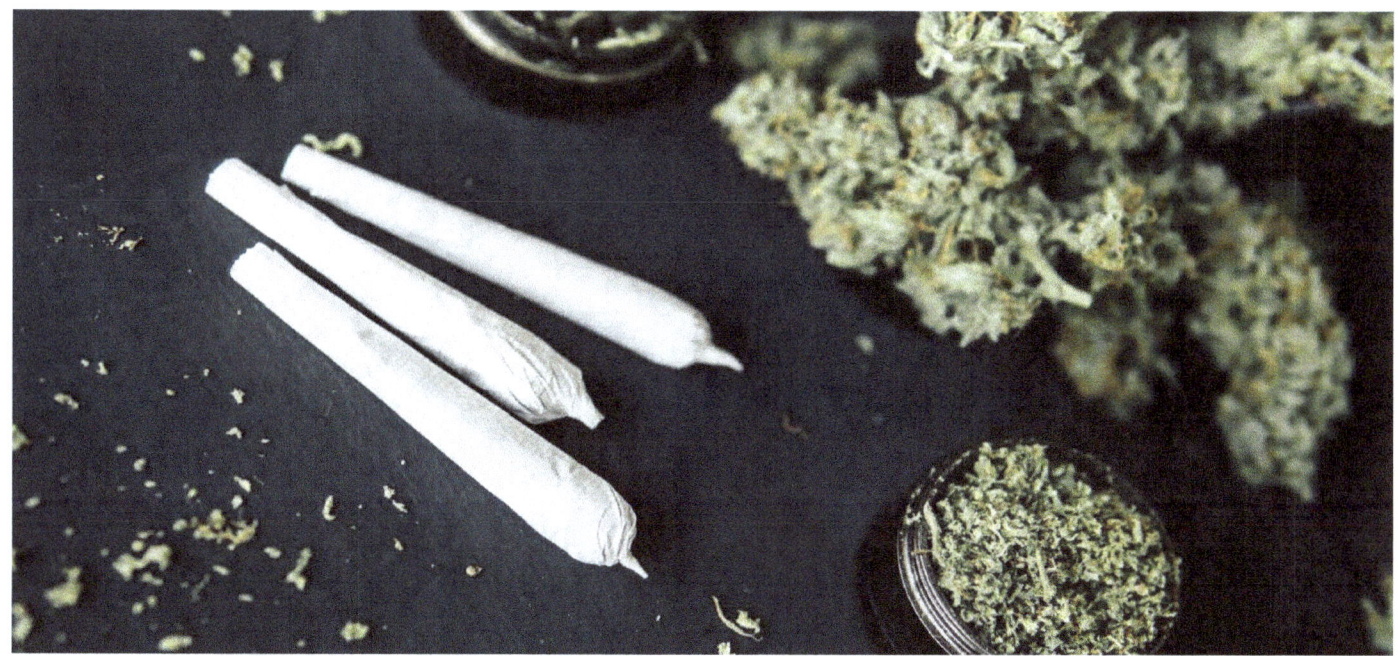

polypharmacy in the population as a whole and across different groups are needed.

A connection between medical cannabis laws and opioid analgesic overdose mortality among individuals who misuse or abuse opioids is less clear. Previous laboratory work has shown that cannabinoids act at least in part through an opioid receptor mechanism and that they increase dopamine concentrations in the nucleus accumbens in a fashion similar to that of heroin and several other drugs with abuse potential. Clinically, cannabis use is associated with modest reductions in opioid withdrawal symptoms for some people, and therefore may reduce opioid use. In contrast, cannabis use has been linked with increased use of other drugs, including opioids; however, a causal relationship has not been established. Increased access to cannabis through medical cannabis laws could influence opioid misuse in either direction, and further study is required.

> **Opioid analgesic overdose mortality continues to rise in the United States, driven by increases in prescribing for chronic pain.** Because chronic pain is a major indication for medical cannabis, laws that establish access to medical cannabis may change overdose mortality related to opioid analgesics in states that have enacted them.

Although the mean annual opioid analgesic overdose mortality rate was lower in states with medical cannabis laws compared with states without such laws, the findings of our secondary analyses deserve further consideration. State-specific characteristics, such as trends in attitudes or health behaviors, may explain variation in medical cannabis laws and opioid analgesic overdose mortality, and we found some evidence that differences in these characteristics contributed to our

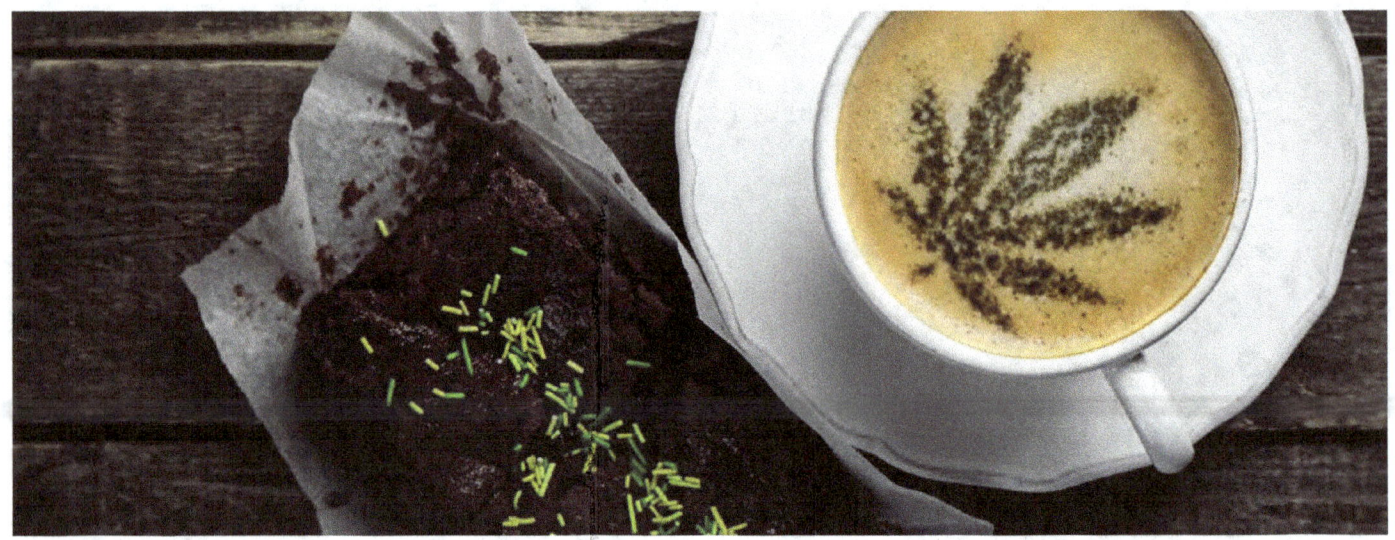

findings. When including state-specific linear time trends in regression models, which are used to adjust for hard-to-measure confounders that change over time, the association between laws and opioid analgesic overdose mortality weakened. In contrast, we did not find evidence that states that passed medical cannabis laws had different overdose mortality rates in years prior to law passage, providing a temporal link between laws and changes in opioid analgesic overdose mortality. In addition, we did not find evidence that laws were associated with differences in mortality rates for unrelated conditions (heart disease and septicemia), suggesting that differences in opioid analgesic overdose mortality cannot be explained by broader changes in health.

In summary, although we found a lower mean annual rate of opioid analgesic mortality in states with medical cannabis laws, a direct causal link cannot be established.
This study has several limitations. First, this analysis is ecologic and cannot adjust for characteristics of individuals within the states, such as socioeconomic status, race/ethnicity, or medical and psychiatric diagnoses. Although we found that the association between medical cannabis laws and lower opioid overdose mortality strengthened in the years after implementation, this could represent heterogeneity between states that passed laws earlier in the study period vs those that passed the laws later. Second, death certificate data may not correctly classify cases of opioid analgesic overdose deaths, and reporting of opioid analgesics on death certificates may differ among states; misclassification could bias our results in either direction. Third, although fixed-effects models can adjust for time-invariant characteristics of each state and state-invariant time effects, there may be important time- and state-varying confounders not included in our models. Finally, our findings apply to states that passed medical cannabis laws during the study period and the association between future laws and opioid analgesic overdose mortality may differ.

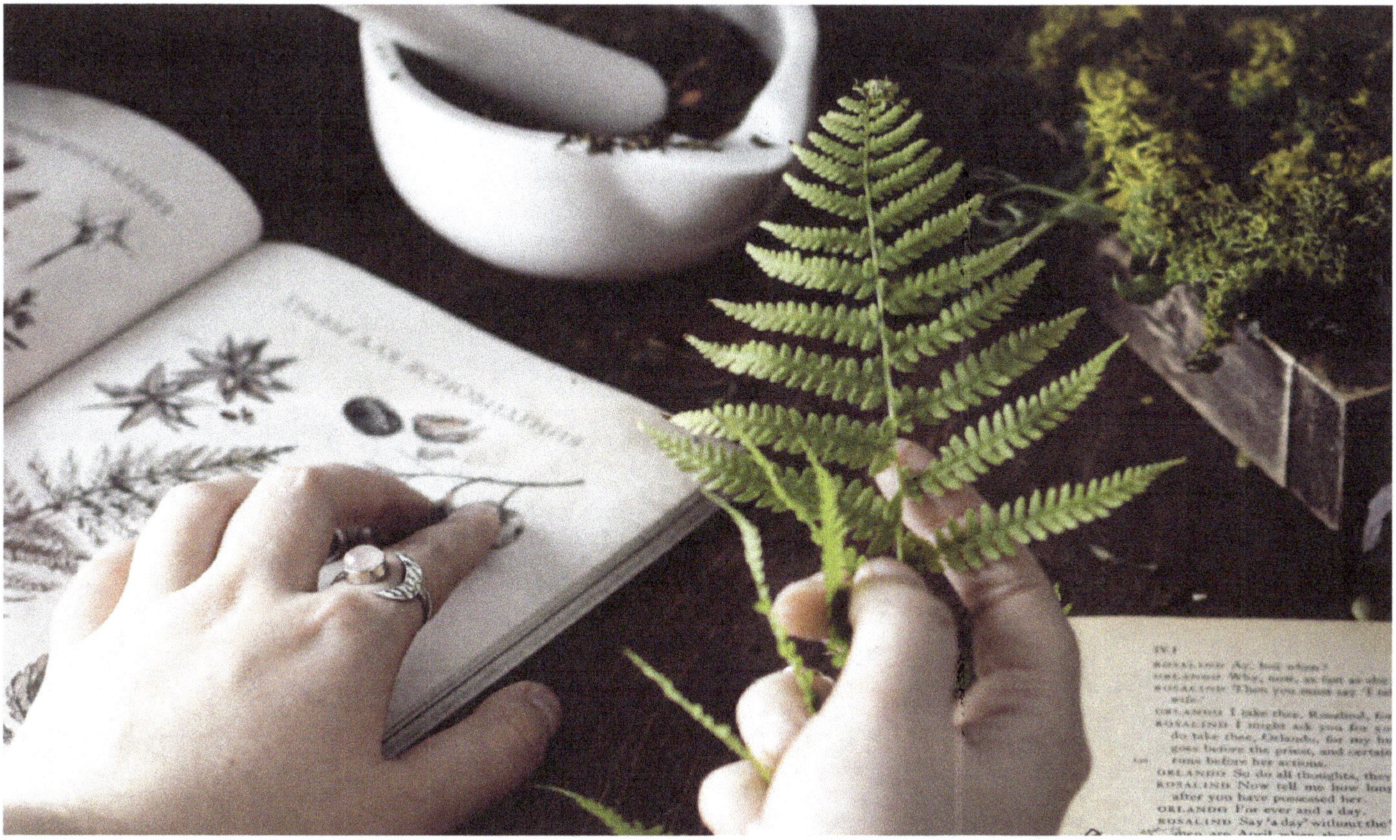

Fern

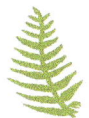

The remains of a medieval skeleton has shown the first physical evidence that a fern plant could have been used for medicinal purposes in cases such as alopecia, dandruff and kidney stones.

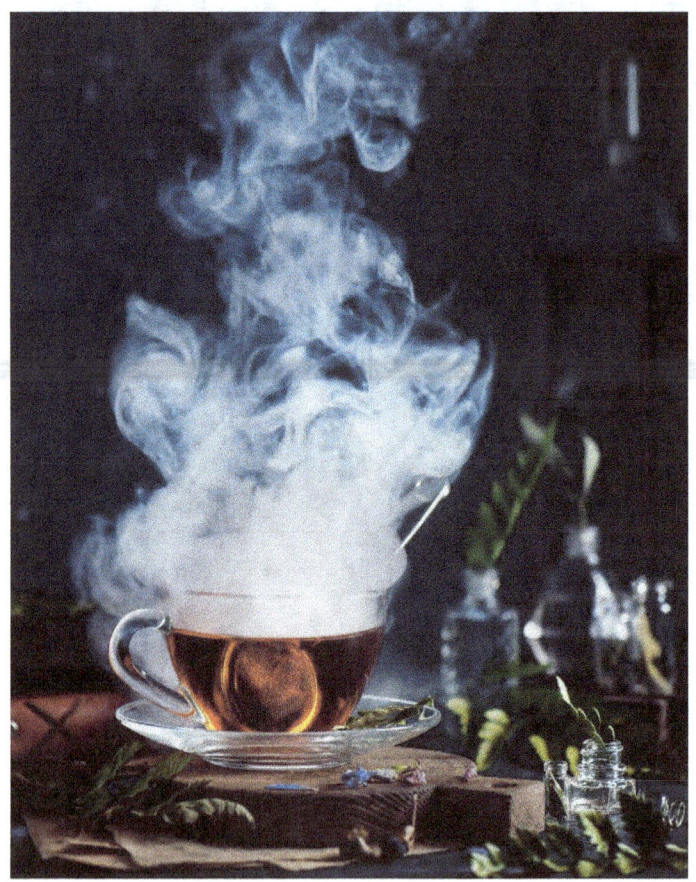

The skeleton of a male aged between 21 and 30 years found buried in the medieval necropolis of Can Reiners on the Spanish Balearic Islands, had traces of starch grains consistent with cereal plants, such as wheat and rye, and significantly, a collection of cells in which spores are formed from the underside of a fern leaf.

There is no evidence to suggest that the fern leaf was part of human diets at any point in recorded history, but there are written descriptions dating as far back as the first century AD that suggest the fern leaf was used to alleviate the symptoms of particular non-life-threatening conditions. Folk medicine stories collected in various books suggest that the fern was used across Europe, but this is the first time any evidence has been found in actual human remains and the first time the particular species of fern has been identified.

Dr Elena Fiorin, from the University of York's Department of Archaeology, said: "Through analysis of the dental calculus of the skeleton, which we believe dates back to the ninth or 10th century, we were able to determine that the cells were from fern plant, asplenium trichomanes, a common species that grows in rocky areas worldwide.

"These ferns have been used by herbalists, surgeons, doctors, and other healers for centuries across Europe, but until now we have only had written documents that describe their use.

"The finding from the dental remains of this skeleton show just how much information we can get from dental calculus analysis. It demonstrates that in this region of Spain, communities were aware of the medicinal properties of some plants and how to administer them to get the desired result."

Records show that a liquid infusion was made by pouring water into fresh or dried fern leaves, and sometimes the concoction was flavoured with orange flowers or sweetened sugar or honey.

> **Herbal texts show that the plants were exclusively used to cure particular diseases, most commonly what we would recognise as dandruff, a common cold, kidney stones, and alopecia.**

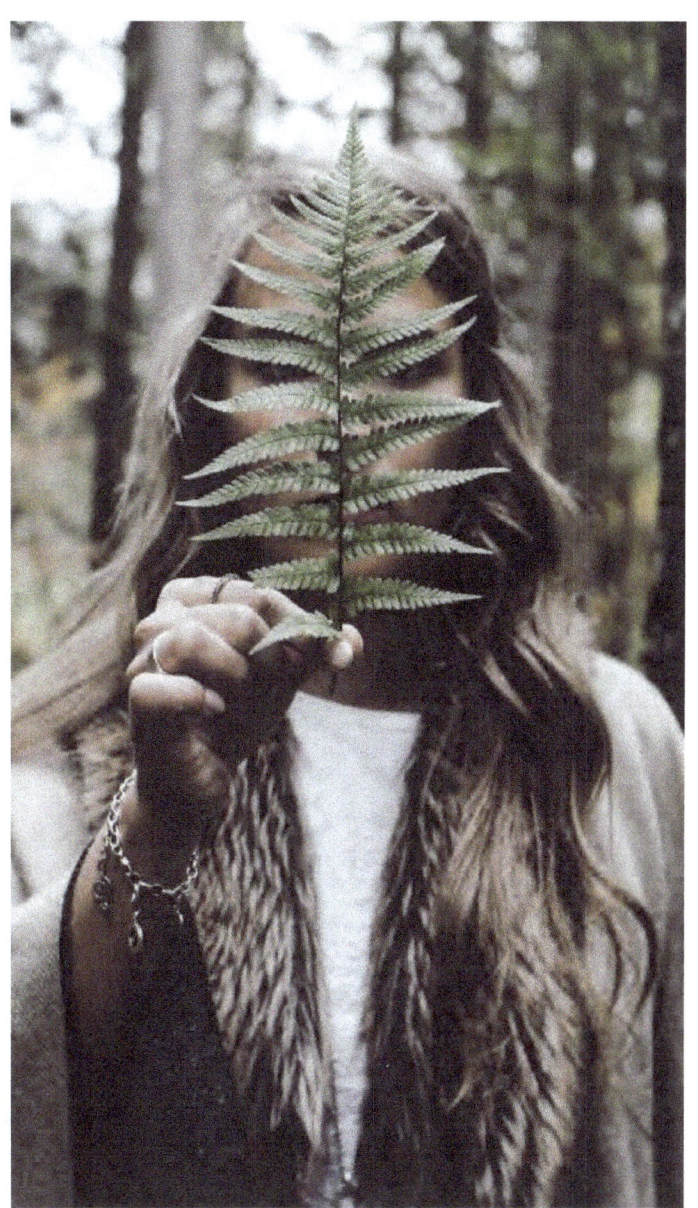

Herbal texts show that the plants were exclusively used to cure particular diseases, most commonly what we would recognise as dandruff, a common cold, kidney stones, and alopecia. There is also reference to the plant being used to stimulate menstrual flow in women.

Although there is no way of telling from the skeletal remains of the young male what he was treated for, it is likely he drank a fern leaf infusion to potentially cure a condition of the skin, urinary tract, or as a decongestant.

Dr Fiorin said: "The research demonstrates the use of ferns as healing plants in the Mediterranean during the Middle Ages. We now have the potential to look at other dental remains for similar properties that might tell us more about the use of medicinal herbs in the past.

"These ferns were employed, and are still used in Europe today, to cure a variety of diseases and through the archaeological record we can start to see how human beings have used the natural environment to assist in healthcare throughout our evolution."

4 Most Common Ferns:

- **Maidenhead - Adiantum pedatum -** Grows in North America and East Asia.

- **Rattlesnake Fern (Botrychium virginianum) -** United States, in the mountains of Mexico, in Australia, in some parts of Asia, as the Himalaya Mountains, and is found also in Norway, in the Karelia region of Finland and Russia, and around Gulf of Bothnia, although in no other part of Europe.

- **Ostrich Fern (Matteuccia struthiopteris)-** Also known as fiddlehead ferns or shuttlecock fern, is a crown-forming, colony-forming fern. It grows in temperate regions of the Northern Hemisphere in central and northern Europe, northern Asia, and northern North America.

- **Bracken Fern (Pteridium aquilinum) -** Also known as 'eagle fern', Bracken Fern a species occurring in temperate and subtropical regions in both hemispheres. The extreme lightness of its spores has led to its global distribution.

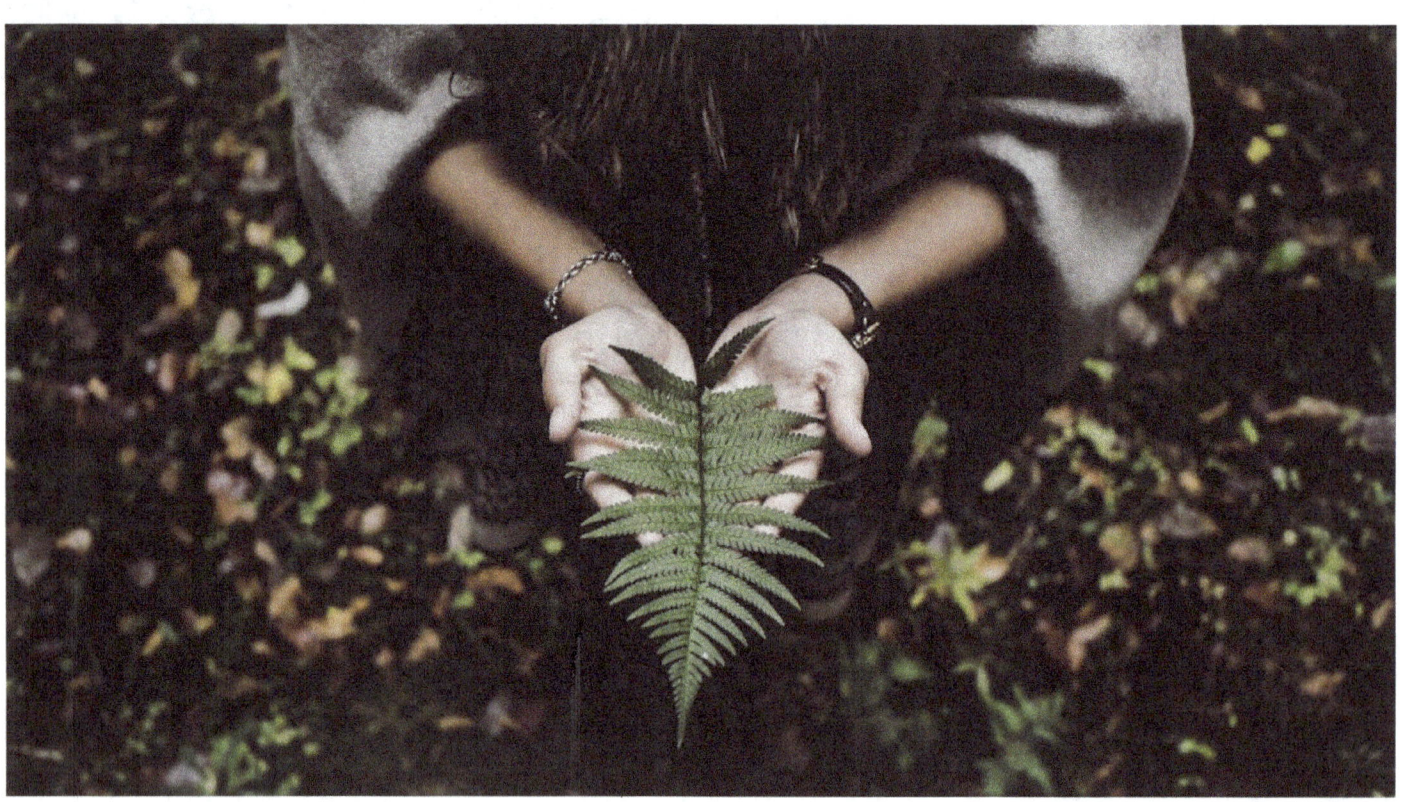

Some Common Ferns uses

- **Maidenhair (Adiantum pedatum)** used for rheumatism.
- **Marginal Wood Fern (Dryopteris marginalis)** used for rheumatism.
- **Sensitive Fern (Onoclea sensibilis)** used for arthritis.
- **Cinnamon Fern (Osmunda cinnamomea)** used externally for rheumatism and internally for joint pain.
- **Christmas Fern (Polystichum acrostichoides)** used for rheumatism.
- **Bracken Fern (Pteridium aquilinum)** used for rheumatism.
- **Ferns** used for Lungs
- **Maidenhair** smoked for asthma.
- **Maidenhair Speenwort (Asplenium tricomanes)** used for coughs.
- **Rattlesnake Fern (Botrychium virginianum)** used as a cough medicine for tuberculosis.
- **Hay-scented Fern (Dennstaedtia penctilobula)** used for chills and lung hemorrhages.
- **Rock Cap (Polyopdium virginianum)** used for sore throat, colds, measles, tuberculosis, cough, and lung congestion.
- **Christmas Fern** used for chills, fever, pneumonia, red spots on skin, listlessness, tuberculosis, and hoarseness.
- **Bracken Fern** used for tuberculosis, infections, and chest pain.
- **Ferns** used for Gynecology (including menstrual, postpartum, and breastfeeding)
- **Walking Fern (Asplenium rhizophyllum)** used topically and as emetic for swollen breasts.
- **Maidenhair Speenwort** used for irregular menses and breast diseases.
- **Lady Fern (Athyrium filis-femina)** used for mothers with intestinal fevers and to prevent water breaking.
- **Mountain Wood Fern (Dryopteris campyloptera)** used for disease of the womb.
- **Ostrich Fern (Matteuccia struthiopteris)** used as decoction of sterile leaf stalk base for the expulsion of afterbirth and for back pain.
- **Sensitive Fern (Onoclea sensibilis)** used for infection, blood disorders (blood deficiency, cold in the blood, and others), and to restore the female system after childbirth. Externally used for sores.
- **Cinnamon Fern** used for women's troubles, caked breasts, and malaise.
- **Interrupted Fern (Osmunda claytoniana)** used for weak blood and gonorrhea.
- **Royal Fern (Osmunda regalis)** used for menstrual problems.
- **Bracken Fern** used for weak blood, uterine prolapse, suffering after birth, caked breast, weakness, and headaches.
- **Marsh Fern (Thelypteris palustris)** used as a gynecological medicine.
- **Ferns** used for the Blood
- **Maidenhair** used as a wash or poultice for bleeding.
- **Lady Fern** used for vomiting of blood.
- **Hay-scented Fern** used for lung hemorrhages.
- **Sensitive Fern** used for blood deficiency, cold in the blood, and other blood disorders.
- **Christmas Fern** used for weak blood and toxic blood.
- **Interrupted Fern** used for weak blood.
- **Bracken Fern** used to make good blood after menses or childbirth.
- **Ferns used for Digestion** (including stomach ache and parasites)
- **Mountain Wood Fern** used for stomachache.
- **Royal Fern** used for intestinal worms.
- **Rock Cap** used for stomachaches and cholera.
- **Bracken Fern** used for diarrhea, nausea and vomiting, infections, diarrhea, weakness, stomach cramps, and headaches.
- **Sensitive Fern** used for intestinal troubles.

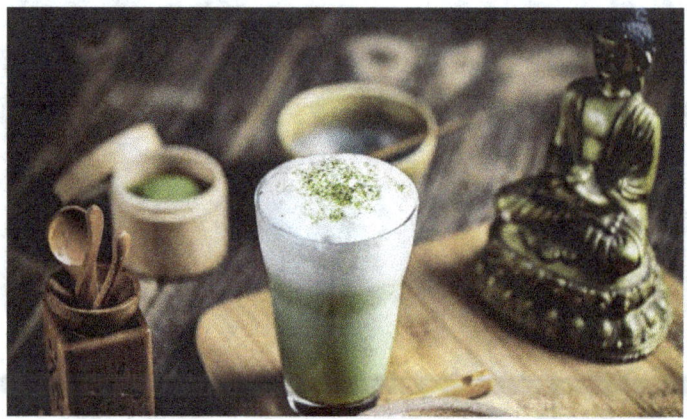

Should you Drink Matcha Tea Regularly

Matcha was the primary way to consume tea in China during the Tang Dynasty (600-900 AD).

Matcha tea comes from the same plant that originates all green, white, and black teas: the camellia sinensis bush. The name "matcha" literally means "powdered tea."

The process of turning tea leaves into a powder is not new. Matcha was the primary way to consume tea in China during the Tang Dynasty (600-900 AD).

In the 1100s, a huge transfer of knowledge and culture from China to Japan occurred, and that's how matcha made its way across the ocean. Matcha and Zen Buddhism flourished together, and the two were often considered inseparable.

By the 1500s, matcha took hold as part of the formal Japanese tea ceremony, which celebrated stillness and simplicity. It grew in popularity in Japan, even as it lost its appeal in China.

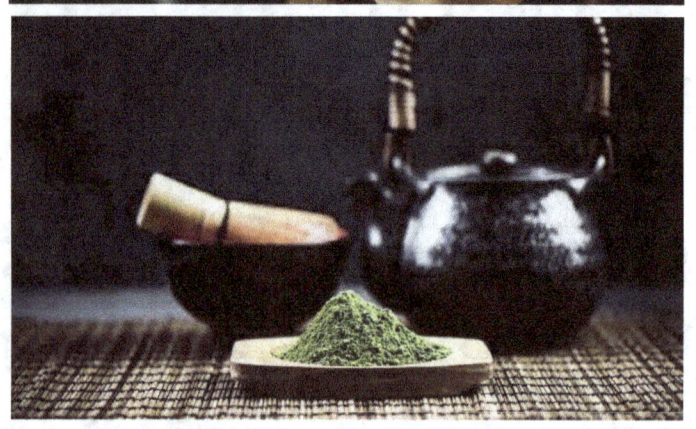

How Is Matcha Tea Different from Regular Green Tea?

We know tea may be the world's healthiest beverage — and green tea seems to be the most healthful of all. But what makes matcha special?

The matcha process begins while the green tea leaves are still growing. The plants are shaded before harvesting to increase chlorophyll and amino acid content (particularly L-theanine) and to improve the appearance and flavor of the tea. This gives matcha powder its brilliant green color.

Once the leaves are harvested, steamed, dried, and blended, they are ground up into a fine powder that you mix into hot or cold water.

The result? You're actually drinking the entire tea leaf! With traditional green tea, in comparison, you're only drinking the dissolvable elements that the leaves infuse into the water.

So matcha powder can give you the health benefits of green tea, and then some! In fact, a cup of matcha tea has about three times the antioxidants of regular green tea.

What Does Matcha Taste Like?

Most people find typical matcha teas have a strong, grassy flavor — similar to wheatgrass or even spinach.
But premium matcha teas have balanced flavors, with layers of unfolding creaminess, umami, fresh-cut grass, and roasted notes.

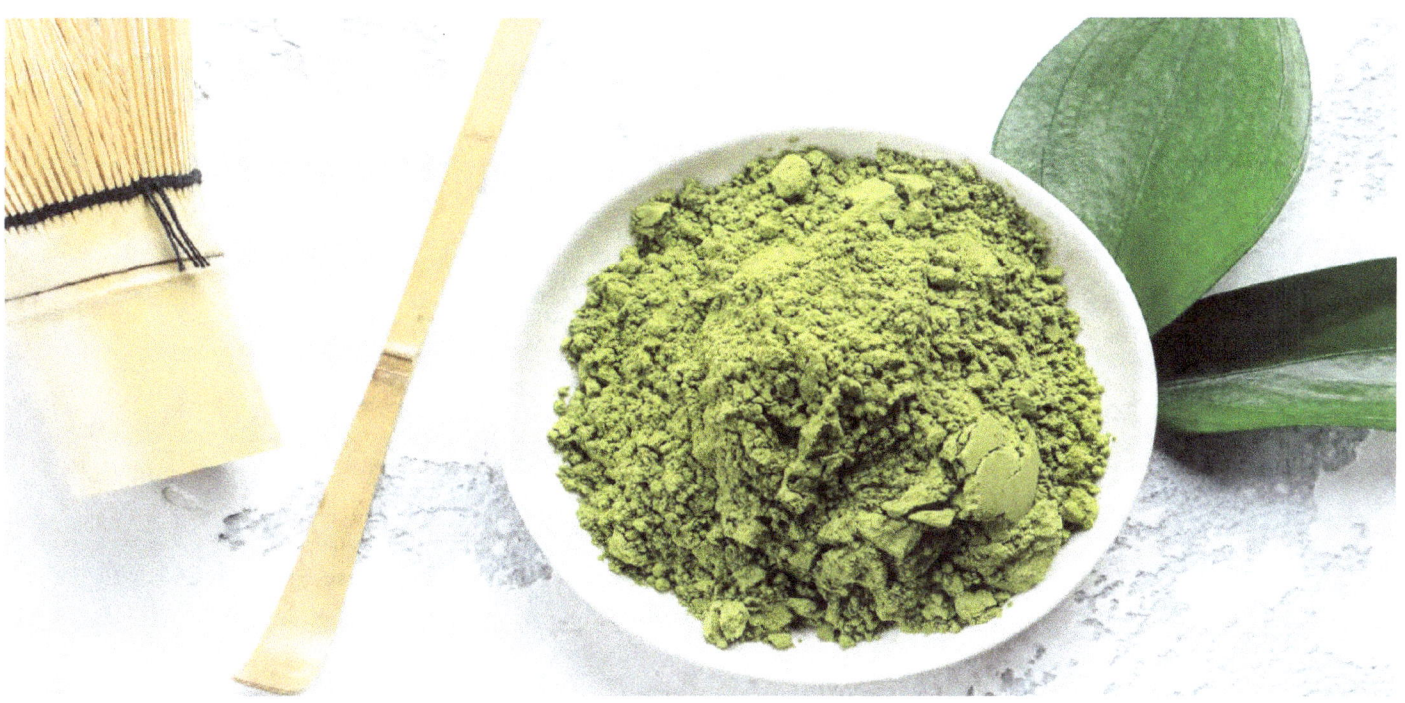

What Are the Benefits of Matcha Tea?

Why might you want to drink matcha? Here are five, science-backed benefits:

1. Supports Heart Health

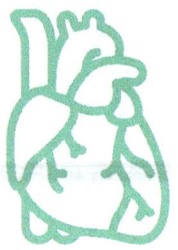

Green tea catechins may support a healthy cardiovascular system. And matcha is the most potent type of green tea when it comes to catechin content.

So where's the evidence for this?

- A 2001 study published in The American Journal of Clinical Nutrition found that "Catechins, whether from tea or other sources, may reduce the risk of ischemic heart disease mortality but not of stroke."
- A meta-analysis of studies on catechins and stroke, published in 2009 in Stroke, however, concluded that "Although a randomized clinical trial would be necessary to confirm the effect... daily consumption of either green or black tea equaling 3 cups per day could prevent the onset of ischemic stroke."

Not only that, a comprehensive analysis published in the American Journal of Clinical Nutrition in 2011 found that "the administration of green tea beverages or extracts resulted in significant reductions in serum TC and LDL-cholesterol concentrations." No effect on HDL cholesterol levels was observed.

Plus the powerful antioxidants found in green tea, especially EGCG, have shown to be helpful in supporting healthy arteries.

2. Supports Healthy Cells

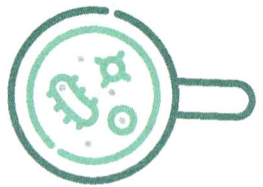

Animal studies suggest that drinking matcha regularly may support your body's natural antioxidant defense system.

This has implications for healthy aging, plus it's excellent news for supporting a stronger immune system!

3. Supports Brain Health

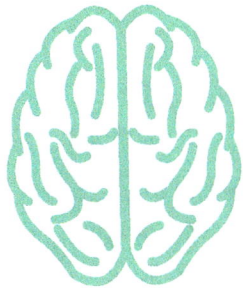

Studies show that consuming matcha can help support healthy cognitive function.

Researchers in a 2014 study published in the journal Nutrients tracked 12 elderly nursing home residents with cognitive dysfunction. They concluded that green tea consumption (in this case, 2 grams of green tea powder — matcha — consumed daily for three months) may be effective in supporting cognitive function, including during aging.

Another 2017 paper published in Food Research International was based on research in healthy adults. The study found that those who consumed matcha exhibited improved performance, suggesting tea may support healthy brain function in young, healthy people as well.

4. Supports Healthy Metabolism

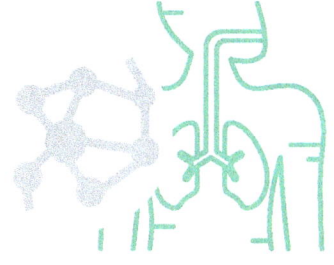

It turns out that matcha may help support a healthy body weight by supporting a healthy metabolism and fat-burning.

In one fascinating 2005 study published in the American Journal of Clinical Nutrition, researchers found that regularly drinking matcha can support elevated thermogenesis (the rate at which you burn calories). The researchers concluded that "Body weight, BMI, waist circumference, body fat mass, and subcutaneous fat area were significantly lower in the green tea extract group than in the control group."

In a 2018 study published in Human Kinetics, women drank a cup of matcha before a 30-minute brisk walk. Scientists learned that consuming the matcha supported fat-burning during the walk.

5. Supports Mood and Mental Focus

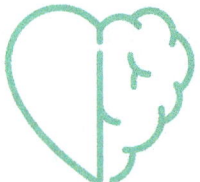

Matcha is rich in amino acids (the building blocks of protein) compared to other teas. And it turns out to be the very highest in one of the most prized amino acids, L-theanine.

What does L-theanine do for you? It can support a calm and meditative state that's perfect for deep focus.

The effect of drinking matcha is commonly described as "relaxed alertness" or "meditation in a cup" because caffeine helps the mind focus and stay alert, while L-theanine helps it relax.

L-theanine is also why the caffeine in tea may not give you the same jitters as the caffeine in coffee does. It acts as a complement to caffeine, balancing the jitters or anxiety you might typically feel, while still providing you with calm energy.

While all green tea contains L-theanine, the levels found in matcha are unmatched. Most green teas have four milligrams of L-theanine per serving, but matcha tea has 20 milligrams!

Even if you're not big on meditating, most of us could do with a little more calm alertness.

Fun fact:
One of the earliest uses of matcha was as an aid to the meditation practice of Japanese monks. Drinking matcha would help them sit alert and calm for hours on end.

Does Quality Matter?
In a word....YES!
Here are five tangible benefits of high-quality matcha teas:
- ♠ Traditionally, the holy grail for great matcha is umami flavor. Umami flavor comes from the high amino acid content. So if you're tasting a lot of umami — the savory flavor of foods such as miso, shiitake mushrooms, and the highest quality soy sauces — you're probably getting a potent dose of amino acids, including calming L-theanine. Highly regarded tea cultivators use a specific method for increasing umami: They shade the tea leaves before harvest to prevent photosynthesis while

overfeeding the plants with nutrients. This enables tea plants to produce and keep a higher level of amino acids, which increases umami flavor.

- The best matcha teas come from the first "flush" or the first pick of leaves in the year during the spring. This is when plants have been resting all winter and produce the most nutrient-dense and flavorful leaves filled with chlorophyll, L-theanine, and catechins. Lower-grade matcha teas are harvested in the summer and fall when plants are fatigued and leaves are less nutrient-dense.
- Higher quality matcha is grown with fewer pesticides and fertilizers, even if they are not organic. (Of course, it's best to go organic, too!) The last thing you want is to increase your exposure to toxins when you drink something you hope could benefit your health.
- Better grinding techniques used to produce high-quality matcha generate less heat, which preserves more nutrients and antioxidants.
- Higher quality matcha teas also just taste better — they are less bitter and grassy. And if you enjoy the taste of something, you're more likely to keep drinking it regularly, right?

Because of the way leaves are grown, shaded, harvested, and processed, the price of matcha reflects the quality. After all, the harvest of high-quality matcha takes place only once each year.

So if you find inexpensive matcha, there's a good chance that the leaves are of a lesser quality without proper processing — which means fewer health benefits. That doesn't mean it's not a good thing. But matcha is one of those things where, more often than not, you get what you pay for.

3 Ways to Choose A Good Matcha Tea

How do you decide which matcha tea is a good one to choose? There are three main ways you can judge a matcha's quality:

- **Flavor —**
  Due to the umami flavor (discussed above), quality matcha teas will have a harmony of creamy, savory, grassy, and roasted flavors.
- **Color —**
  What you want is a beautiful bright and vibrant green. If your matcha is on the yellow side, that means it's of a lesser quality and comes from leaves harvested later in the year instead of during the spring.
- **The Appearance of Froth —**
  The traditional method of drinking matcha involves whisking it with a bamboo whisk to create a frothy foam. If the bubbles are large and irregular, this means the matcha powder is coarsely ground and of lesser quality. The highest quality matcha, on the other hand, is finely ground and creates foam made of tiny, uniform bubbles when whisked with skill.

When Should You Drink Matcha?

Due to its caffeine content, morning or afternoon is the best time to consume matcha.

People with sensitive stomachs may experience discomfort when drinking the tea on an empty stomach due to its tannin content. (Tannins are bitter-tasting but harmless chemicals

that occur naturally in tea and wine.)
If you are one of these people, you might have better results if you wait until after you've had breakfast or lunch to drink your matcha.

Final Word: Should You Try Matcha Tea?
No food or beverage, no matter how many benefits medical studies may find, is right for everyone at all times. Matcha contains caffeine, and not everyone responds well to caffeine. If you find that it doesn't work for you — no problem. You'll find some other fabulous, health-boosting beverages, here. But for many people, quality matcha is worth a try. You can take a little time out of your day to savor the experience and let yourself bask in the rich flavors and calming energy it brings.

After all, we can all enjoy a little bliss now and then.

● Editor's note:

Want An Excellent Matcha Tea? Check This Out
Do you want to drink matcha tea? As you've seen above, selecting a high-quality brand is important — like Pique Tea's Sun Goddess Matcha.

Why is this organically grown matcha tea excellent? It starts with its source. This matcha comes from Kagoshima, the furthest point from industrial pollution and radiation in Japan — and also neighbor to Okinawa, a Blue Zone where natives enjoy the longest lives in the world!

And then, the company quadruple screens for heavy metals and toxins, pesticides, mold, and radioactive isotopes — harmful things you definitely don't want to be drinking in a healthy beverage!

This matcha tea also maximizes its health benefits because the tea leaves are shaded 35% longer to produce more amino acids, including L-theanine.

Not to mention, it has an incredible, creamy, umami flavor that is quite delightful — and is also award-winning.

Lab-Grown Human Skin To Reduce Animal Testing

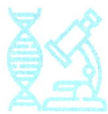

'Upwards of 90 percent of drugs that are proven safe and effective in animals fail during clinical trials'

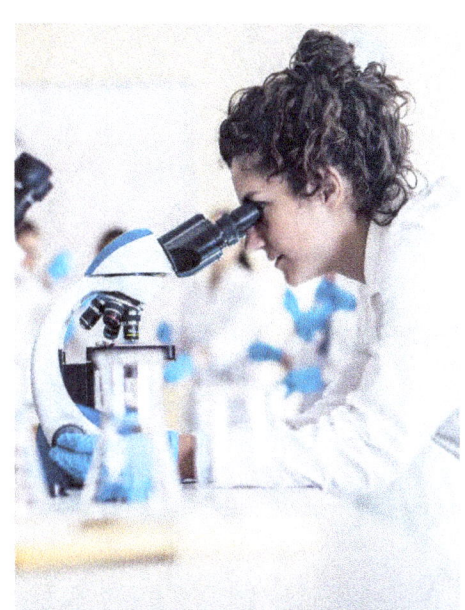

TenSkin is said to 'closely mimic intact, living skin' (Photo: Adobe).

Researchers from the University of Dundee have created lab-grown human skin in an effort to reduce the need for animal testing.

Founded by Dr. Robyn Hickerson and Dr. Michael Conneely, Ten Bio Ltd has developed a product dubbed as 'TenSkin' which is said to 'closely mimic intact, living skin'.

'More effective'

According to The Times, Dr. Conneely said: "The skin that covers our body is under tension, this has been known for a long time.

"Other models don't incorporate this tension, and this is why our product is more effective. When skin is removed from the body it contracts as the tension relaxes." He added that by stretching the skin 'to an optimal tension', the duo have created a model allowing both pharmaceutical and cosmetics companies to 'generate pre-clinical data that will be much more predictive of what is likely to be seen in the clinic'.

'Global cosmetics company'

"While animals can serve as good analogs to study general principles, they often fail when it comes to specific details due to animal/human species differences…" added Dr. Hickerson.

"Upwards of 90 percent of drugs that are proven safe and effective in animals fail during clinical trials."

The company has reportedly signed a contract with a 'global cosmetics company' and is working on launching its website.

Starting a Plant-Based "Eat To Live" Life

One of the most powerful steps you can take to improve your health, boost energy levels, and prevent chronic diseases is to move to a plant-based diet. Science shows changing your nutrition is a powerful way to live longer, help the environment, and reduce your risk of getting sick.

According to the Permanente Journal, Health care professionals, even Holistic ones should invite their colleagues, patients, and their families to a shared decision-making process with the goal of adopting a plant-based diet and a regular exercise program. We should invite health care teams to complete a course on healthy eating and active living. We should encourage staff to be knowledgeable about plant-based nutrition. Finally, we should encourage performance-driven measurable outcomes, which may include:

1. The percentage of patients in a physician panel with high blood pressure, diabetes, high cholesterol, or cardiovascular disease who completed a course on nutrition that emphasizes a plant-based diet.

Too often, physicians ignore the potential benefits of good nutrition and quickly prescribe medications instead of giving patients a chance to correct their disease through healthy eating and active living. If we are to slow down the obesity

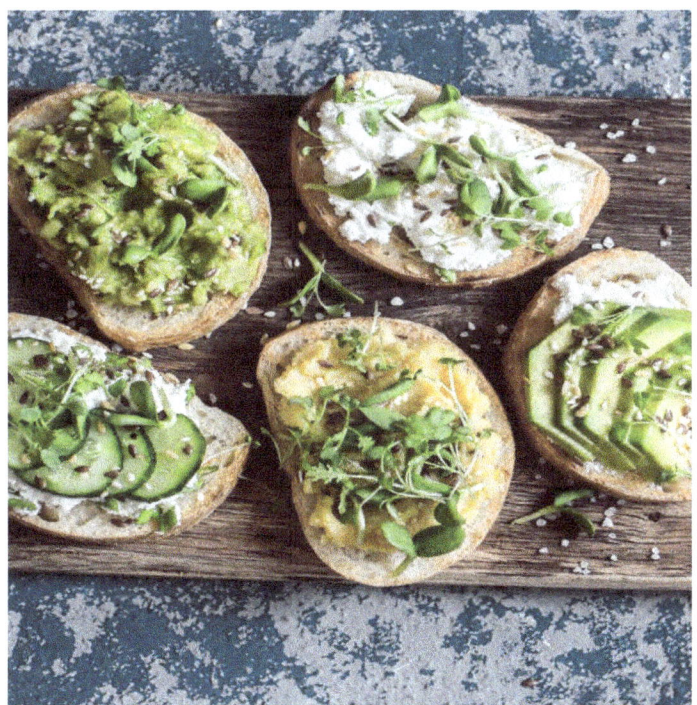

> You're probably thinking that moving to a plant-based diet sounds like a great idea, but you don't know where to start. Don't worry, we have a list of grains—easy and enjoyable. We'll provide tips you might need.

epidemic and reduce the complications of chronic disease, we must consider changing our culture's mind-set from "live to eat" to "eat to live." The future of health care will involve an evolution toward a paradigm where the prevention and treatment of disease is centered, not on a pill or surgical procedure, but on another serving of fruits and vegetables. However, we must evolve and begin our plant-based journey as a society.

How A Whole-Food, Plant-Based Diet Can Boost Your Health

There's excellent scientific evidence that many chronic diseases can be controlled, reduced, or even reversed by moving to a whole-food, plant-based diet. Scientific research highlighted in the landmark book The China Study shows that a plant-based diet can reduce the risk of type 2 diabetes, heart disease, certain types of cancer, and other major illnesses. Many people also report bigger fitness payoffs, more energy, reduced inflammation, and better health outcomes after making the switch.

What Is A Whole-Food, Plant-Based Diet?

A whole-food, plant-based diet is based on the following principles:

- **Whole food** describes natural foods that are not heavily processed. That means whole, unrefined, or minimally refined ingredients.
- **Plant-based** means food that comes from plants and doesn't include animal ingredients such as meat, milk, eggs, or honey.

A whole-food, plant-based diet lets you meet your nutritional needs by focusing on natural, minimally-processed plant foods.

The Benefits Of Discovering Transitions Foods, For a Plant-Based Diet

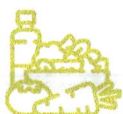

"I get a lot of questions about how to transition to a plant-based diet. I know it can be overwhelming when you're just starting out but I want to assure you that you can do this. It might be hard at first and most likely you'll stumble along the way but all that matters is that you keep trying."

I've been eating this way for so long, sometimes I forget what it's like to come from the opposite end of the spectrum. If you've been eating a heavily animal-based diet, the transition to a plant-based diet might seem impossible. You might be thinking what could one possibly eat if you don't eat meat, eggs and dairy? Well, don't you worry. I'm here to assure that not only is there plenty of nourishing, delicious foods to eat but they can be prepared as fun and creative plant-based alternatives to all your favourite foods.

50/50 Diet

Just remember when transitioning it is better to incorporate 2 oz. of meat into your daily diet as you transition. We call this the 50/50 diet where we have 50% vegetables and 50% non-vegetables.

Change Your Mindset

It's important to approach this new chapter with an open mind and a positive mindset. Try to think in terms of what you'll be gaining from eating a plant-based diet instead of what you'll be missing out on. Maintaining your new diet shouldn't be about willpower, struggle or deprivation. In fact, once you learn more about plant-based eating, you'll see that don't have to give anything up.

Once you're familiar with the ins and outs of vegan alternatives to pizza, cookies, muffins, chocolate and sandwiches, you'll have no problem learning to love the plant-based lifestyle and how it makes you feel.

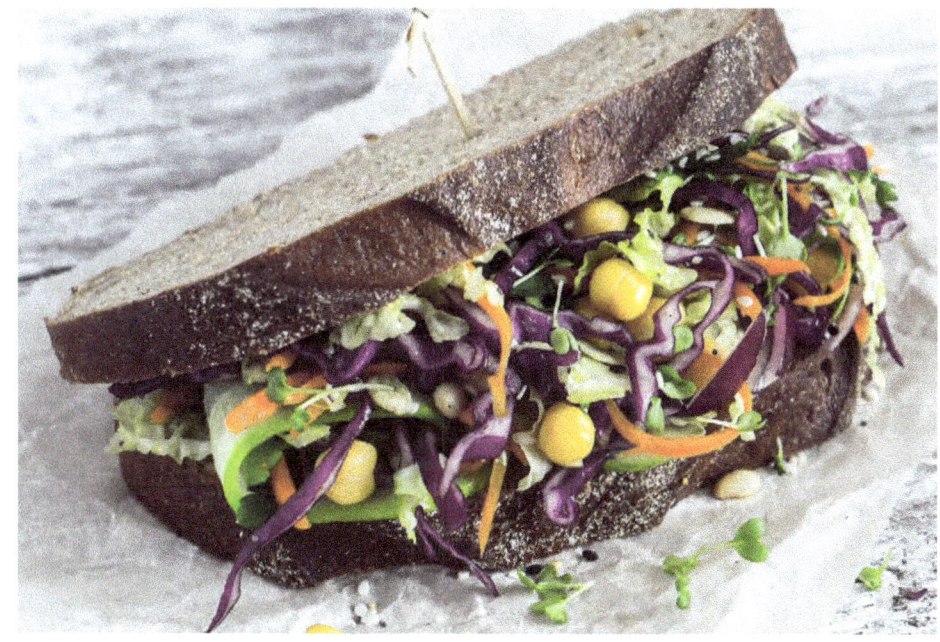

> Having a well-stocked pantry of essentials will simplify your shopping lists and allow you to create healthy and delicious meals on the fly. **Check out my post on How to Stock a Vegan Pantry to get started.** You may also find my vegan grocery list helpful, grab a copy below.

Know Your Reason Why

It's important to get really clear on your reason for embarking on a whole food plant-based diet. If it's a big lifestyle change for you, it's going to get tough at times and having a clear reason why can help you stick to your goals.

Reasons for eating plant-based could include:

- preventing disease
- managing blood sugar
- lowering cholesterol
- living longer
- love for animals
- losing weight
- reducing your environmental impact

There are a lot of great reasons to eat a plant-based diet. What one speaks to you? Find a reason that inspires you and get really clear on it. Write down your why and stick it on your fridge or bathroom mirror. Keep that reason front and center to help you stay focused.

Prepare Your Own Food

This is probably the most important aspect of eating plant-based. Unless you have unlimited funds for food and live somewhere with tons of vegan restaurants, preparing your own food at home is absolutely key to making a whole food plant-based diet work. So it's time to get in the kitchen! There's no need to spend hours cooking, creating healthy plant-based meals can be quick and simple.

Meal Plan And Food Prep

I recommend doing at least some food prep every week. It will make your life so much easier, save you money and prevent food waste. I would also recommend sitting down on Sundays and completing a meal plan and grocery list. Planning and preparation and key to success.

Once you have a plan for the week and a complete grocery list, it's time to shop and then get in the kitchen to do some food prep. This could be as simple as pre-washing and chopping all your veggies, or as thorough as batch cooking all your meals for the week. Experiment and see what works for you.

Stock Your Pantry
Having a well-stocked pantry of essentials will simplify your shopping lists and allow you to create healthy and delicious meals on the fly. Check out my post on How to Stock a Vegan Pantry to get started. You may also find my vegan grocery list helpful, grab a copy below.

Educate Yourself
This step is huge too. The more you learn about health, nutrition, animal welfare and agriculture, the easier making plant-based choices becomes. I would recommend checking out my list of plant-based diet resources at the back of this magazine.

Pick Up Some New Cookbooks
I like using my favourite vegan cookbooks for ideas when I'm doing my weekly meal planning. Check out the Media Guide at the back of the magazine for some of my Favorite plant-based cookbooks.

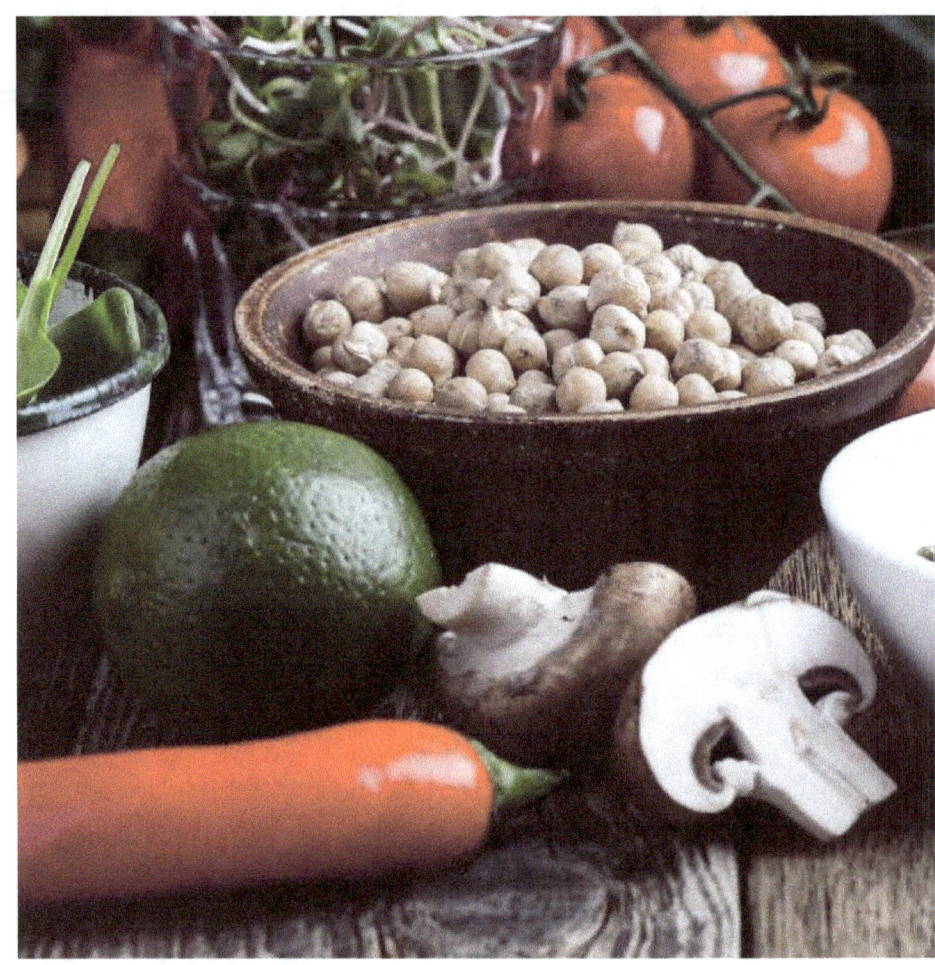

Your Whole-Food, Plant-Based Diet—
The Foods You'll Love

There are plenty of other foods you can also enjoy— including nuts, seeds, tofu, tempeh, whole-grain flour and breads, and plant-based milks.

Here's a quick overview of the major food categories you'll enjoy on a plant-based diet, with examples:

Fruits: any type of fruit including apples, bananas, grapes, strawberries, citrus fruits, etc.

Vegetables: plenty of veggies including peppers, corn, avocados, lettuce, spinach, kale, peas, collards, etc.

Tubers: root vegetables like potatoes, carrots, parsnips, sweet potatoes, beets, etc.

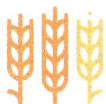

Whole grains: grains, cereals, and other starches in their whole form, such as quinoa, brown rice, millet, whole wheat, oats, barley, etc. Even popcorn is a whole grain.

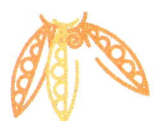

Legumes: beans of any kind, plus lentils, pulses, and similar ingredients.

There are plenty of other foods you can also enjoy— including nuts, seeds, tofu, tempeh, whole-grain flour and breads, and plant-based milks. However, we recommend eating these foods in moderation, because they are more calorie-dense and can contribute to weight gain.

How To Transition To A Plant-Based Diet

If you're currently eating closer to the Standard American Diet, working in stages towards a completely plant-based diet is probably your best bet for success.

Transitioning to a plant-based diet doesn't have to be done cold turkey. Your transition might take 4 weeks and it might take a year, so don't expect perfection or to get there overnight. Change can be difficult and it can be emotionally and socially challenging to break free from the norm. Depending on where you're at in your healthy eating journey, you may be able to make the switch right away but for those of you with a bigger change to make, a slow transition might be the way to go.

Transitioning In Stages

If you're currently eating closer to the Standard American Diet, working in stages towards a completely plant-based diet is probably your best bet for success. One step at a time. This will make it realistic and sustainable as you're bound to stumble along the way until you find your footing and eating plant-based starts to come naturally.

There's no need to feel pressured to get to a fully plant-based diet overnight. The journey is all part of the fun, so if you can learn to love the process you'll be much more likely to succeed in the long term.

Step 1.
Start Reducing Your Meat Consumption.

If you're brand new to all this, start going meatless once per week. Meatless Mondays is a popular movement so that could be a good day to start with. I would recommend incorporating Meatless Mondays into your routine for 2-4 weeks before moving on.

If you currently eat eggs, fish and dairy, don't worry about that yet, just focus on incorporating more plant food into your diet and eating less meat. Instead of making meat the star of your dishes, try making a bean, legume or tofu-based dish or making that side salad the main course.

Start Adding More Plants

While you're transitioning in the first month, not only do you want to start eliminating meat but it's also time to start adding more plant-based foods to your diet. For example, if you normally eat scramble eggs for breakfast, try adding spinach, mushrooms and onions to the mix.

If you're eating soup, stir in some chickpeas and kale, if you're making a sandwich, try adding avocado and sprouts. By adding plant-based foods, you'll also be adding tons of healthy fibre and nutrients plus the more plant foods you eat, the less you'll need animal products and processed foods. During this month you can also focus on trying new foods and recipes and start developing on your weekly food prep and planning habit.

Step 2.
Reduce Meat Consumption Down To Once A Week.

Now that you've got the hang of what one day of plant-based eating is like, it's time to start reducing your meat consumption down day by day until you're only eating it about once a week. You can stay in this second stage for another month or two until you're ready

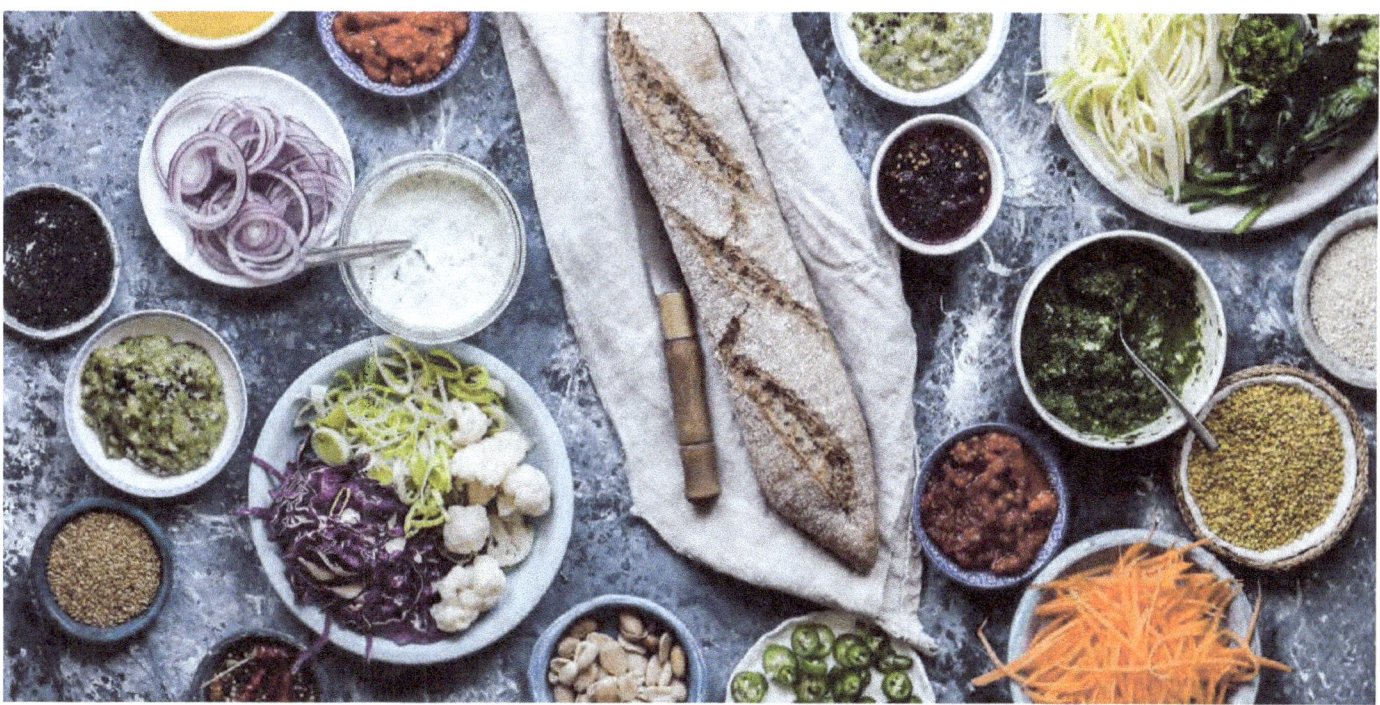

to cut meat down to once every couple of weeks and then once a month.

Step 3.
Eliminate Meat From Your Diet.
It's time! Moving from a 50/50 plan to a complete plant-based diet. You've been moving towards a plant-based diet for at least a month now. You're familiar with how to create a meal plan, food prep and create a full day worth of plant-based meals. So what are you waiting for? At this time, it can help to review your why, check back in with some plant-based nutrition books and podcasts to help keep those big reasons in front of mind. You got this!
If you've been 2 oz of meat or eating fish, it's now time to reduce and then eliminate that as well.

Step 4.
Start Reducing Your Dairy Intake.
A lot of people struggle with cutting out dairy but once you get the hang of it, it's easier than you think. Head over and read my post on How to Replace Dairy in Your Diet to get started.

Replace Cow's Milk First
Milk is the easiest. There are a ton of plant-based milks on the market today and and making your own is easy. Dairy-free milks can be used as a direct replacement for dairy milk and it's an easy switch to make. Do it now.

Then The Yogurt
Yogurt is easy too. You can make your own cashew, almond or coconut yogurt or go for one of the many wonderful store-bought options such as So Delicious or Yoso.

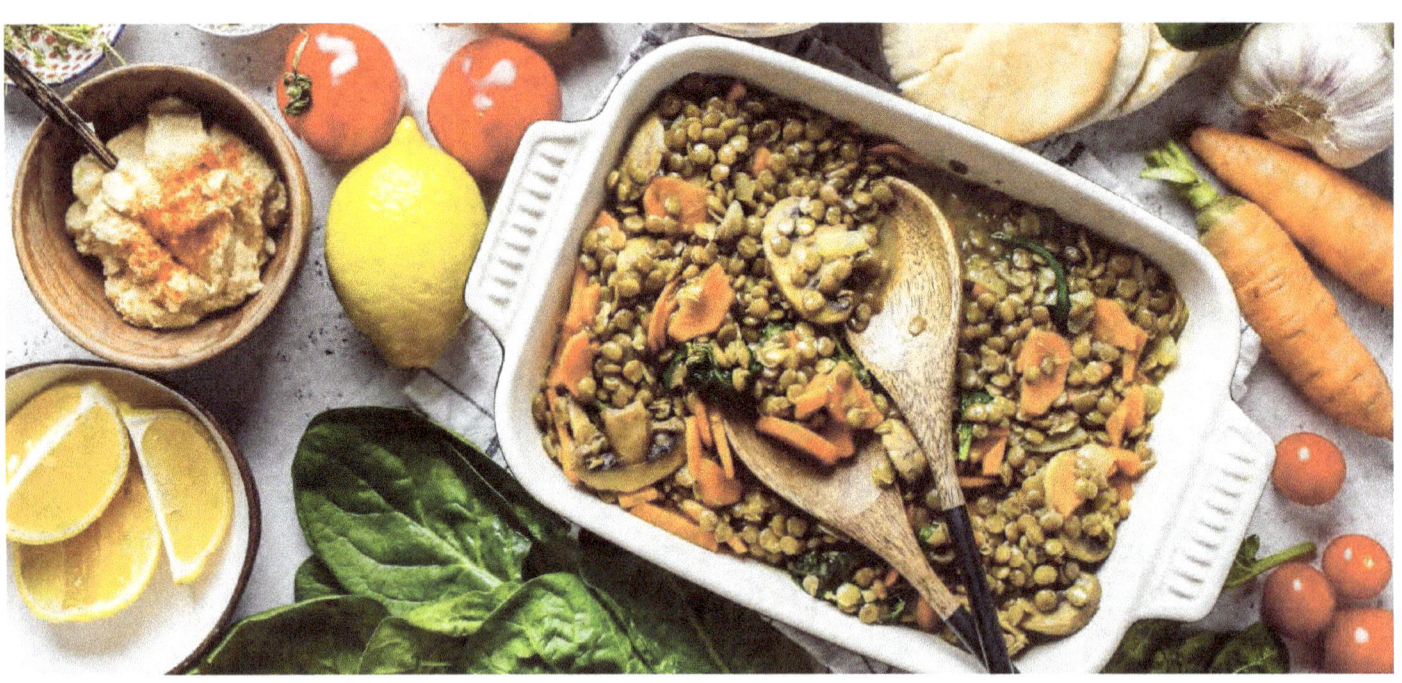

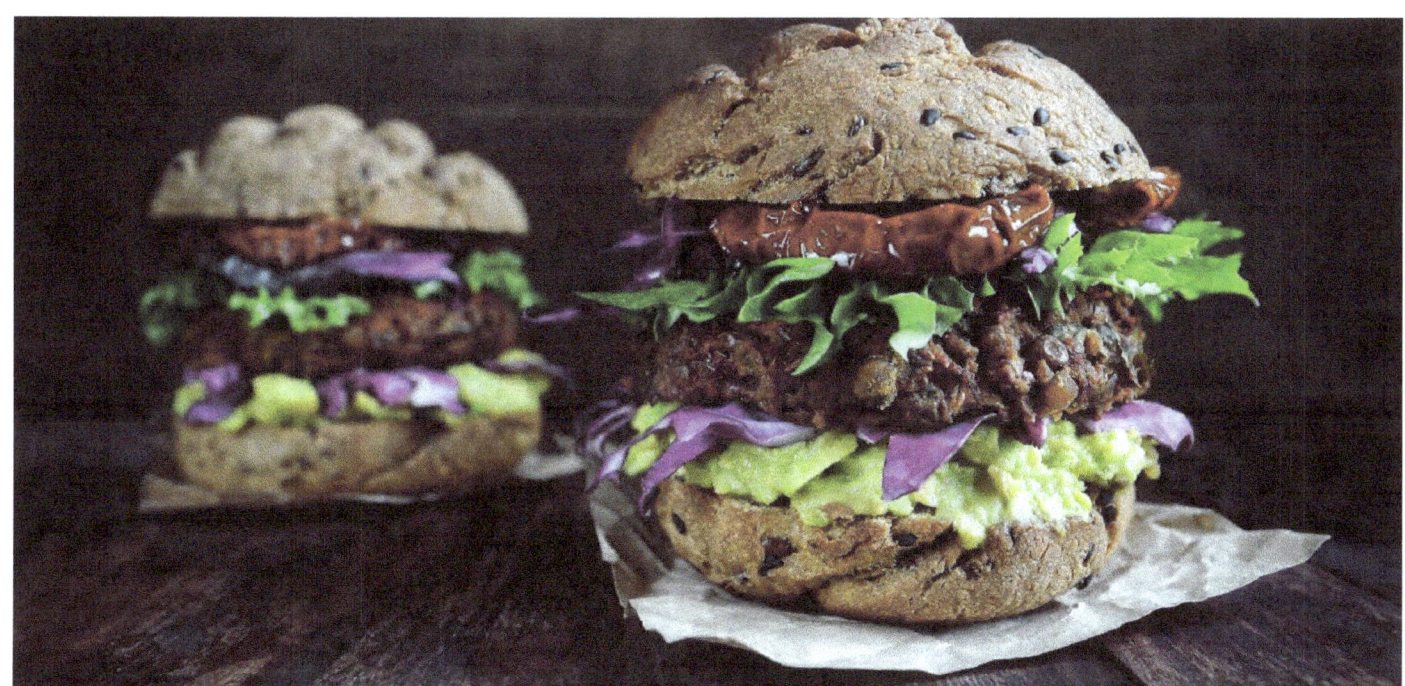

Then The Cheese

Next is cheese. This is probably the hardest for most people since it's hard to replicate the way cheese melts however, at some point you just have to go for it. You will get used to living without cheese. I would suggest listening to this podcast episode: Rich Roll Podcast Episode #2 with Dr. Neal Barnard, On Breaking the Dairy Addiction. There are also a ton of incredible vegan cheeses on the market today. Chao, Daiya and Earth Balance are my favourite larger brands. You can also make your own vegan cheeses, check out This Cheese is Nuts by Julie Piatt if you're interested in homemade plant-based cheeses.

Lastly, The Dairy "Extras"

Next is things like cream, cheese sauce, sour cream and whipped cream and these are all easy to replace with homemade or store-bought vegan alternatives. Get friendly with ingredients like soft tofu, cashews and coconut milk and you'll be able to create your own version of these traditionally dairy-based products.

Spend a few weeks experimenting with plant-based options to replace dairy. Swap out your dairy-milk for almond or cashew, get familiar with nutritional yeast, try making vegan sour cream with cashews or tofu, try tofu ricotta, try making vegan coffee creamer, replace mayonnaise with vegan mayo or avocado and try a few store-bought vegan cheeses if you want to make a treat like pizza or nachos.

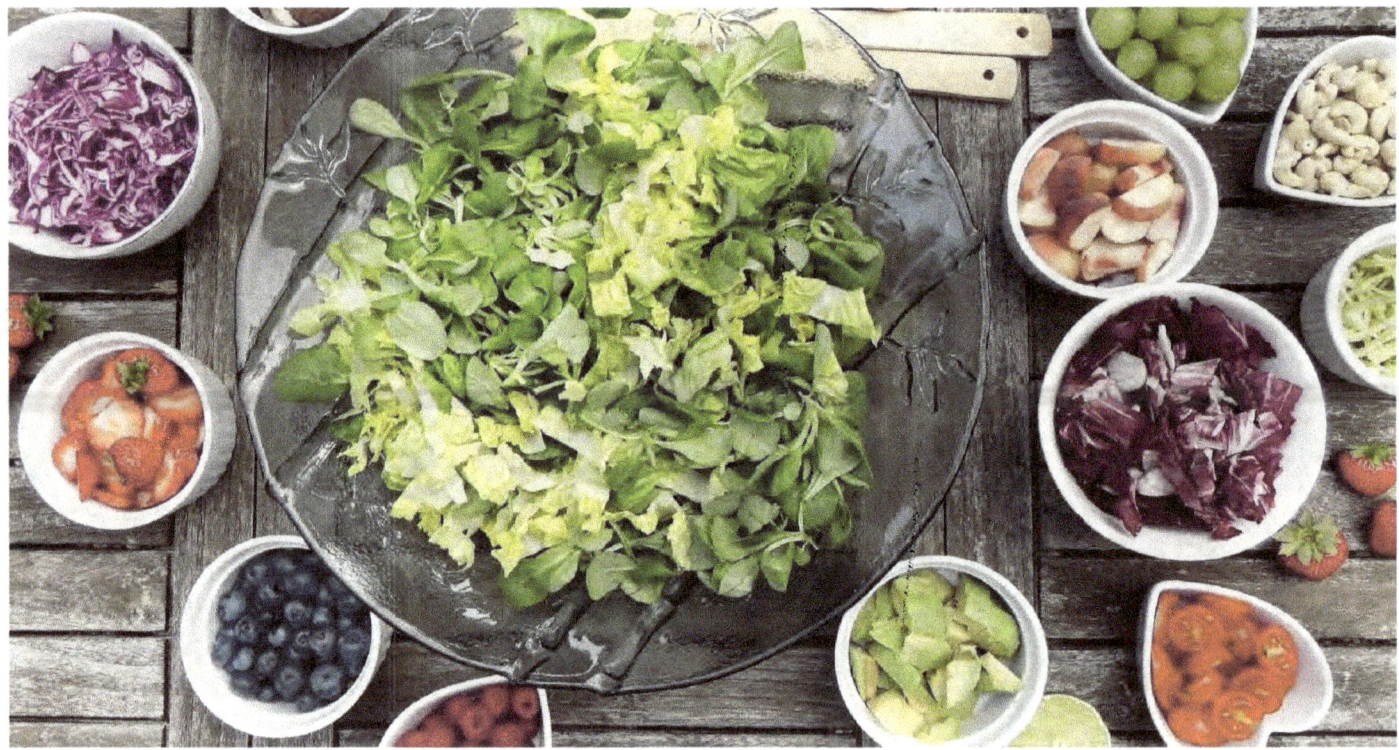

Step 5.
Eliminate Dairy From Your Diet.
Okay, so you've been spending some time familiarizing yourself with vegan alternatives to dairy. It's time to cut it out completely. I'd take a week or two here adjusting to living dairy-free.

Step 6.
Start Reducing Your Egg Intake.
I know some people are reliant on eggs, especially at breakfast time but hopefully you've already been experimenting with plant-based breakfasts. If you normally eat eggs at breakfast time, start reducing that day by day and incorporating new breakfast options such as:

Step 7.
Eliminate Eggs From Your Diet.
Okay, the final step. Cutting out eggs. You've already cut out meat, fish and dairy and you should be almost completely plant-based. You've spent the last few weeks trying vegan breakfast options and replacing eggs in any baking you might have done, so it's time to take that last step and go for it.

Step 8.
Repeat For Life!
Depending on how your journey went, it may have been a week, a month or 6 months since you started. Either way, at this point, you should be completely

plant-based! Congratulations! Now, repeat that for life. Continue exploring new foods, cuisines and recipes. Keep learning, go easy on yourself and just enjoy this amazing, plant-based lifestyle.

Do I Have To Eat Plant-Based Forever?

Do you have to be 100% plant-based for you entire life? That's up to you but the short answer is no, of course not. It's your body, your health and your decision, so do what's right for you and just remember that it's the little things we do consistently over time that matter the most.

Develop Supporting Healthy Habits

Health is more than just what we eat. Stress management, exercise and fun all play a roll. Now is a good time to start incorporating more healthy habits that will support your nutrition plan. These aspects of healthy living can be integrated into your routine at any time. They seem simple but they all play a roll in holistic living so you can feel your best and live life to the fullest.

- **Drink more water.**

Hydration is just as important as nutrition. Drink a lot of water, starting with a big glass first thing in the morning and then continuing throughout the day, it's as simple as that.

- **Meditate.**

Study after study has shown the positive benefit of meditation. This can be as simple as 5 minutes of deep breathing with your eyes closed. Anything to just slow down for a moment and notice what's happening inside and around you. I use the Insight Timer and Calm apps to meditate, Headspace is also very popular.

- **Exercise. Move a lot.**

You'll feel better, look better, live longer, have more energy, sleep better... the list goes on. It doesn't mean you have to go crazy in the gym every day or run mile after mile but it is important to break a sweat and stay active on a daily basis.

- **Journal.**

Journalling is a great way to de-stress, reduce anxiety, focus on goals, create a strong vision for your life and just a good way to chill and become more aware of how you're feeling.

- **Read.**

It's been said the fastest way to improve your life is to read at least 30 minutes a day.

- **Spend time in nature.**

- **Try new things.**

Keep your brain sharp by challenging it with new experiences on a consistent basis.

- **Improve your sleep.**

Look for Tips for Better Sleep and How to Optimize Your Sleep and start making quality sleep a priority.

- **Play, laugh and have fun.**

Laughter really is the best medicine. Play with your kids, go to a comedy show, play games and find ways to bring more play into your days.

- **Create connections.**

Whether it's spending screen-free time with family and friend to getting out and connecting with your community. Human connection and a sense of belonging have been shown to be a key contributor to happiness and longevity.

....

"

There are a ton of plant-based milks on the market today and and making your own is easy. **Dairy-free milks can be used as a direct replacement for dairy milk** and it's an easy switch to make.

....

The Benefits Of A Whole-Food, Plant-Based Diet

> People who eat a plant-based diet tend to be leaner than those who don't, and the diet makes it easy to lose weight and keep it off—without counting calories.

There are several major benefits to moving to plant-based nutrition, all supported by excellent science. These benefits include:

- **Easy weight management:**
People who eat a plant-based diet tend to be leaner than those who don't, and the diet makes it easy to lose weight and keep it off—without counting calories.

- **Disease prevention:**
Whole-food, plant-based eating can prevent, halt, or even reverse chronic diseases, including heart disease, type 2 diabetes.

- **A lighter environmental footprint:**
A plant-based diet places much less stress on the environment.

Who could say no to rice rolls, Spanish quinoa, or a Buddha bowl? You can easily experiment with giving some of your own favorite recipes a plant-based makeover. Replace the meat in your favorite chili with beans or lentils, cook up some wonderful veggie burgers, or make vegetables the star attraction in that stir fry instead of chicken.

Plant-Based Eating Faq?

We know that a sudden shift to plant-based eating isn't for everyone. We asked one of our expert contributors, Craig McDougall, MD, for his advice: "Add around 1,000 calories of legumes, whole grains, and starchy vegetables to your everyday routine. These starchy foods keep you full and satisfied, so you'll naturally eat less of the animal products and processed foods that are making you sick." Dr. McDougall has plenty of other great advice to share.

We encourage people to "not sweat the small stuff" and to look at the big picture instead: "Focus on the big changes like switching from meat, milk, and eggs to whole plant foods. Such changes dramatically improve the nutritional composition of your diet, so this is where you will find the most noticeable and measurable improvements in your health."

The time to start making the change is now. You'll be glad you did.

How Do I Know If A Whole-Food, Plant-Based Diet Is For Me?

You don't—until you try it! So many people who make the switch report feeling much better, having less fatigue, and losing weight, and otherwise enjoying a healthy lifestyle. We make the switch super easy with our extensive tools and resources.

Once you get started, it'll be easier to keep going. As Dr. Craig McDougall says, "Once you have more energy, have lost some weight, or your stomach pain has disappeared, then it's easier to continue eating healthfully. One of the best motivators for people transitioning to plant-based eating comes from how great they feel and how much more they can do in their lives once they're feeling healthier."

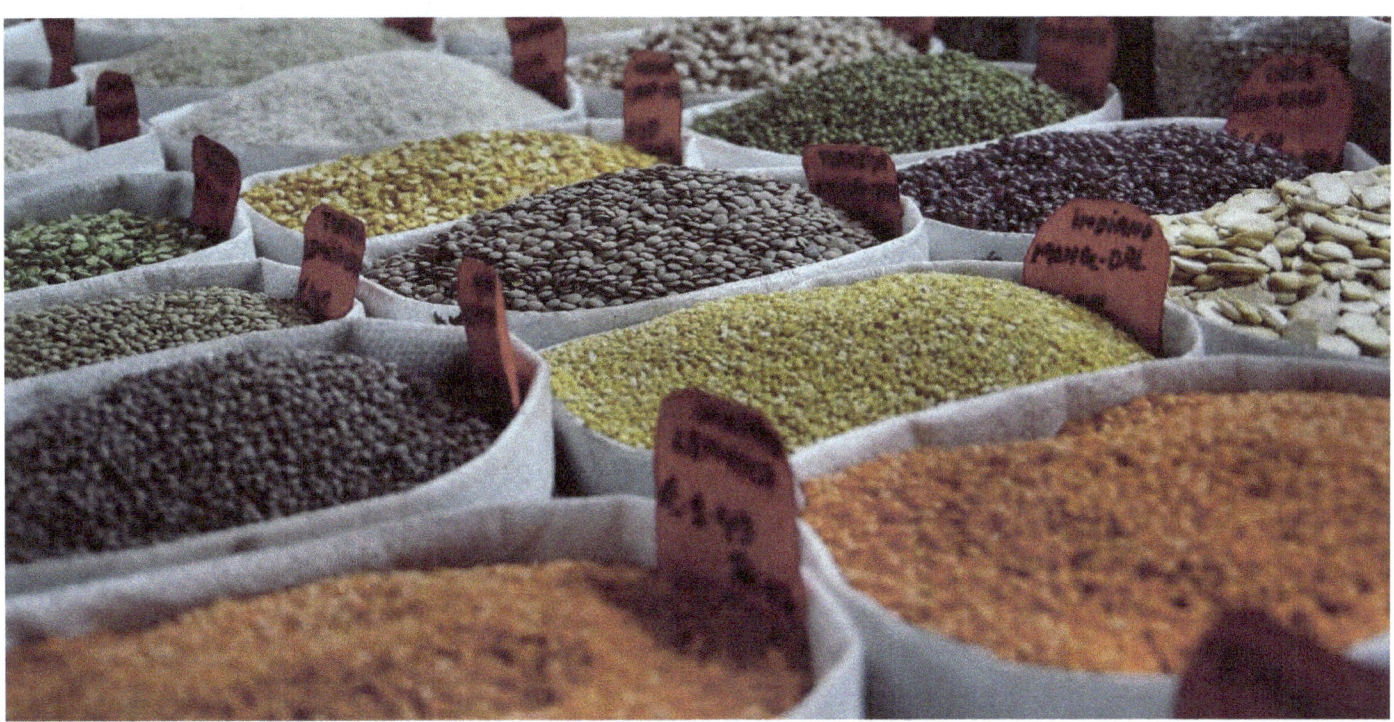

Can I Eat A Plant-Based Diet On A Budget?
Whole-food, plant-based eating is cheaper than you think. Fresh produce goes a long way, and whole grains, potatoes, and beans are some of the most affordable bulk foods you can buy. Create meals around these staple items and you'll definitely spend less than you do on a diet rich in meat and other animal products.

How Can I Eat Whole-Food, Plant-Based While Traveling Or Away From Home?
You will need to plan ahead a little, but it's pretty easy to find whole-food, plant-based meals on the go. You can usually find fruit and dishes made with pasta, rice, and potatoes wherever you are. With a little creativity and flexibility, you can also prepare some fantastic food to take with you.

How Do I Eat Out On A Plant-Based Diet?
Most restaurants are very accommodating of dietary needs, and you should be able to review their menu online. Scan the menu in advance to see if a restaurant offers vegan options, and you're already most of the way there. When you're unsure, simply call ahead, explain your preferences, and they will probably be able to accommodate you.

How Do I Make Sure I Get The Nutrients I Need?
Whole plant foods contain all the essential nutrients (with the exception of vitamin B12) we need. You can get some B12 from fortified foods such as plant-based milks and breakfast cereals, but the best source is a simple B12 supplement. (In fact, the U.S. Department of Health and Human Services recommends supplemental B12 for all adults over age 50 because as we age, many people lose the ability to absorb vitamin B12 from food sources.)

Start Your Journey Today

I hope that helped clear some things up so you can get started on your plant-based journey. Remember, there is power in small change. Take things one day, one step, one meal at a time if you have to and watch those small steps compound into big changes.

Health is a lifelong journey. Start now, don't give up, you got this!

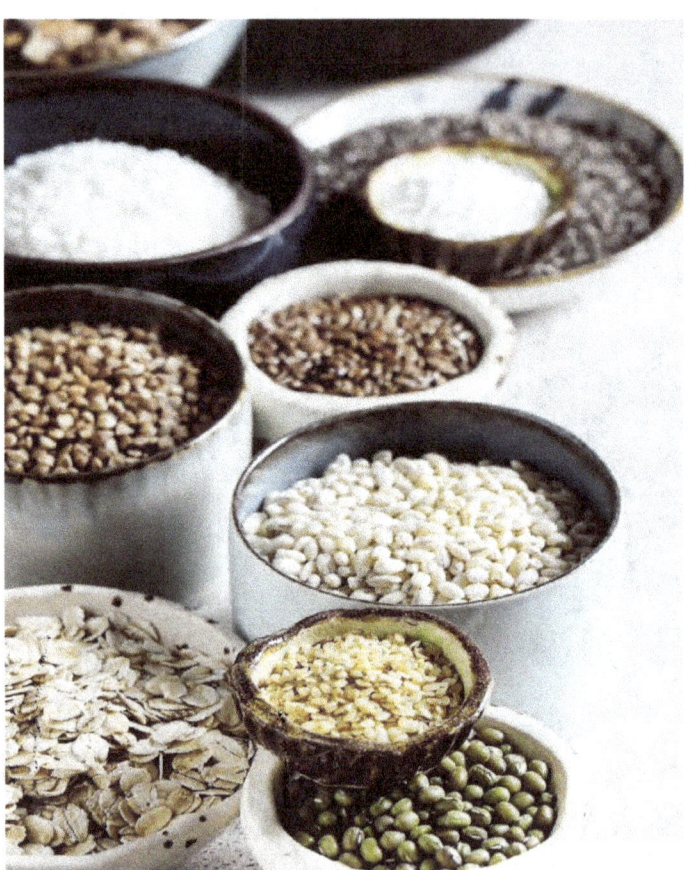

Healing with hemp: Glow Holistic's Farm

Cannabidiol, or CBD, is another ingredient in hemp. CBD is extracted from the hemp plant and, in Glow Holistic's case, is used to make health products.

Before starting Glow Holistic in 2018, Benjamin Clark and his wife Eunice wanted nothing to do with cannabis products. It wasn't until friends of his parents in North Carolina started growing hemp that Clark, after extensive research, said he recognized the crop's benefits.

After leaving his job as a mate with the Jamestown Ferry, he began to grow and sell hemp at his farm in King William County last year.

"We weren't looking to get into this at all — to me cannabis was bad, it always has been," Clark said. "... I looked into it, and the more research [I did] about it, and the benefits of CBD and how it's helping people, we decided to get into it.

"At that same time, Virginia was talking about opening up its VDACS program last year. The timing really worked out quite wonderfully for us."

Hemp, like marijuana, is derived from the Cannabis sativa plant, but its level of tetrahydrocannabinol, or THC, is much lower — usually less than 0.3% — and the plant can be used in various industries, including agriculture, construction and, historically, shipbuilding.

Cannabidiol, or CBD, is another ingredient in hemp. CBD is extracted from the hemp plant and, in Glow Holistic's case, is used to make health products.

Peter Grinspoon, contributing editor for Harvard Health Publishing, notes that CBD has been used successfully to treat epilepsy in children and is also used to treat anxiety and sleep-related issues.

Archaeology report of City Farm gives insight into past occupants For the Clarks, their tinctures, balms, creams and gummies have been about healing others.

"We're amazed at the feedback from people, that it helps them with so many different things, from sleeping and problems sleeping to people with cancer that are taking it and all different things," he said.

In January 2018, Virginia bills HB532 and SB247 were first introduced. They became law July 2018 and allowed the commissioner of the Virginia Department of Agriculture and Consumer Services to lead research through the creation of two different programs.

One program was designated for research by institutions of higher education, while the other is for state research. The creation of the state's industrial hemp research program meant farmers did not have to pair up with a university to grow hemp plants. Glow Holistic was the third business in the state to get its registration from VDACS last year, according to Clark. President Donald Trump signed off on the Farm Bill in December 2018, which addressed a variety of agricultural issues and legalized the industrial production of hemp nationwide. In March 2019, Gov. Ralph Northam signed off on a new amendment to the Industrial Hemp Law, which mirrors regulations set for hemp by the Farm Bill. The amendment allows for commercial growing, with no restrictions on what growers do with the hemp they grow. Even with the expanding legislation, Clark says navigating hemp regulations has not been easy.

"The state and federal government are kind of issuing different regulations at the same time, and so they sort of conflict," Clark said. "There's a lot of

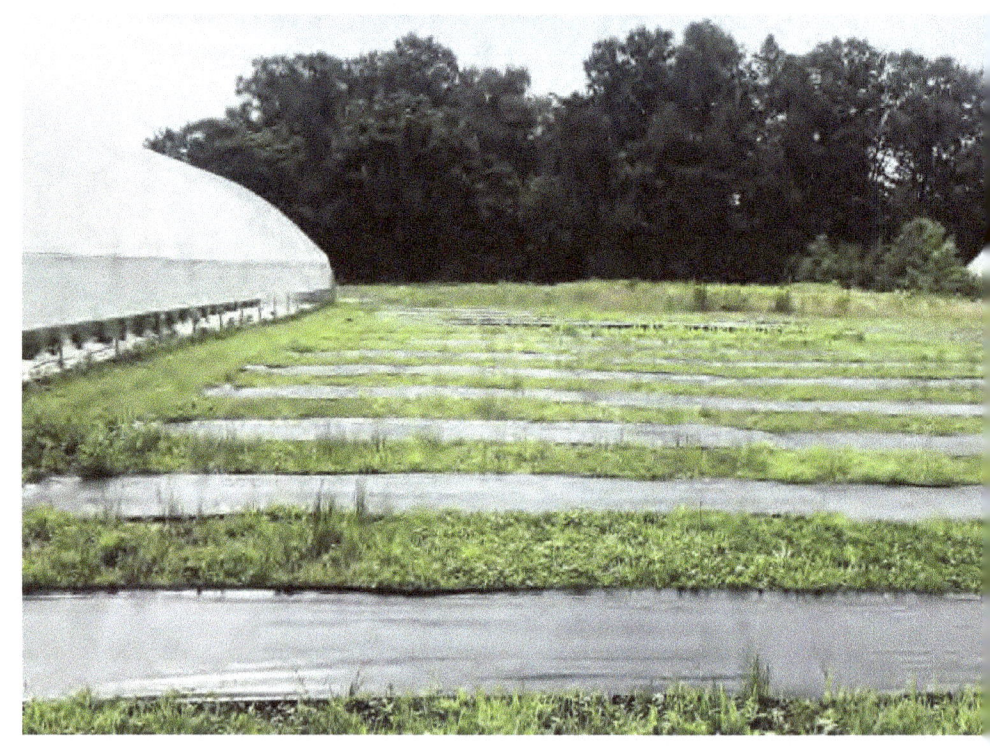

interest [in hemp], and that's good. But at the same time, the industry is moving so rapidly that the legislation is not able to keep up."

Glow Holistic sells its products on its website, at West Point Pharmacy, King William Pharmacy and at a few places in Williamsburg. They also display their products at 2nd Sundays and collaborate with alternative health service Tasha's Own to produce CBD oil-infused goat's milk soap. Eunice Clark said it's important for those who sell CBD products to accurately disclose how many milligrams of CBD is in the product and to price those products appropriately.

"There was one time we went to Virginia Beach and they had a bath bomb and it only had 14 milligrams and they sell it for $12," she said. "Ours has 200 milligrams, and we're going to sell it for $15. We want [customers] to have that and not just baloney."

The couple manages 2 acres with two greenhouses, an irrigation field for outdoor plants and a drying room. The greenhouses' light uses a long-day schedule, allowing for year-round production and crop yields three times a year instead of once.

'We know that people are still struggling': House of Mercy continues to serve Williamsburg community amid pandemic »

The final version of the hemp is packaged and stored in the dry room before being sent off to extractors so the plant's CBD oil can be cultivated. Glow Holistic does not do extraction in-house because the needed machinery is expensive, Clark said.

While Clark will look into expansions for Glow Holistic, such as a new dry room facility, he said he is grateful for the support they have had from the community.

"We really feel blessed and happy to be part of something that is helping people," he said. "It's something that is really changing the quality of life for people."

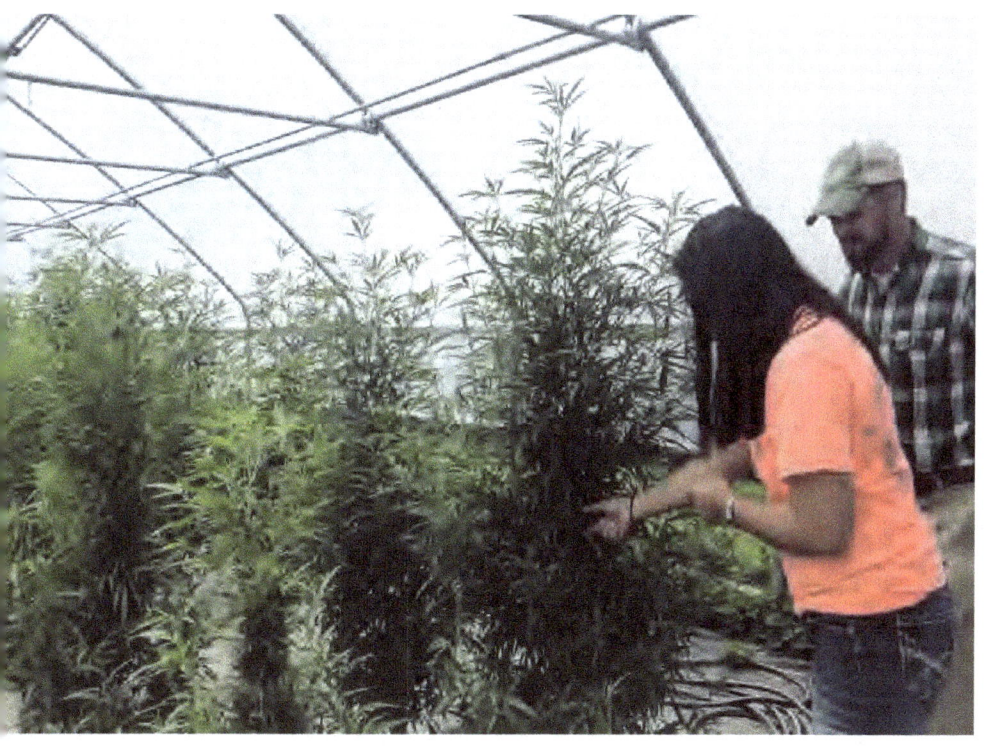

The Basic Principles Of **Therapy**

Every person's soul remains pure and intact. And good. Abuse and harm – all forms of distortion – can only occur in the channels that connect the soul to conscious or subconscious experience.

1. Problems are never what they seem to be. Aggravation and upsetness is never for the reasons people say or even think.

2. Interpersonal difficulties originate in interpersonal ones.

3. The root of all conflicts is the dichotomy between body and soul.

4. The subjective self is unable to totally rise above itself to discover the true root of his/her issues. One needs an objective and intelligent observer to help him examine himself (the necessary criteria for an observer, see below #10).

5. Every human being was created independent; a self contained entity with a unique role. In the image of G-d who is one and indivisible.

6. Every person's soul remains pure and intact. And good. Abuse and harm – all forms of distortion – can only occur in the channels that connect the soul to conscious or subconscious experience. The difference between people is not in their having a soul but in their awareness of it.

7. Everyone has the capacity to access their unscarred soul. Everyone must assume responsibility for themselves (rather than blame another for their problems). The help they need is only in accepting that responsibility and unraveling the distortions and resulting confusion, and charting a course toward positive growth.

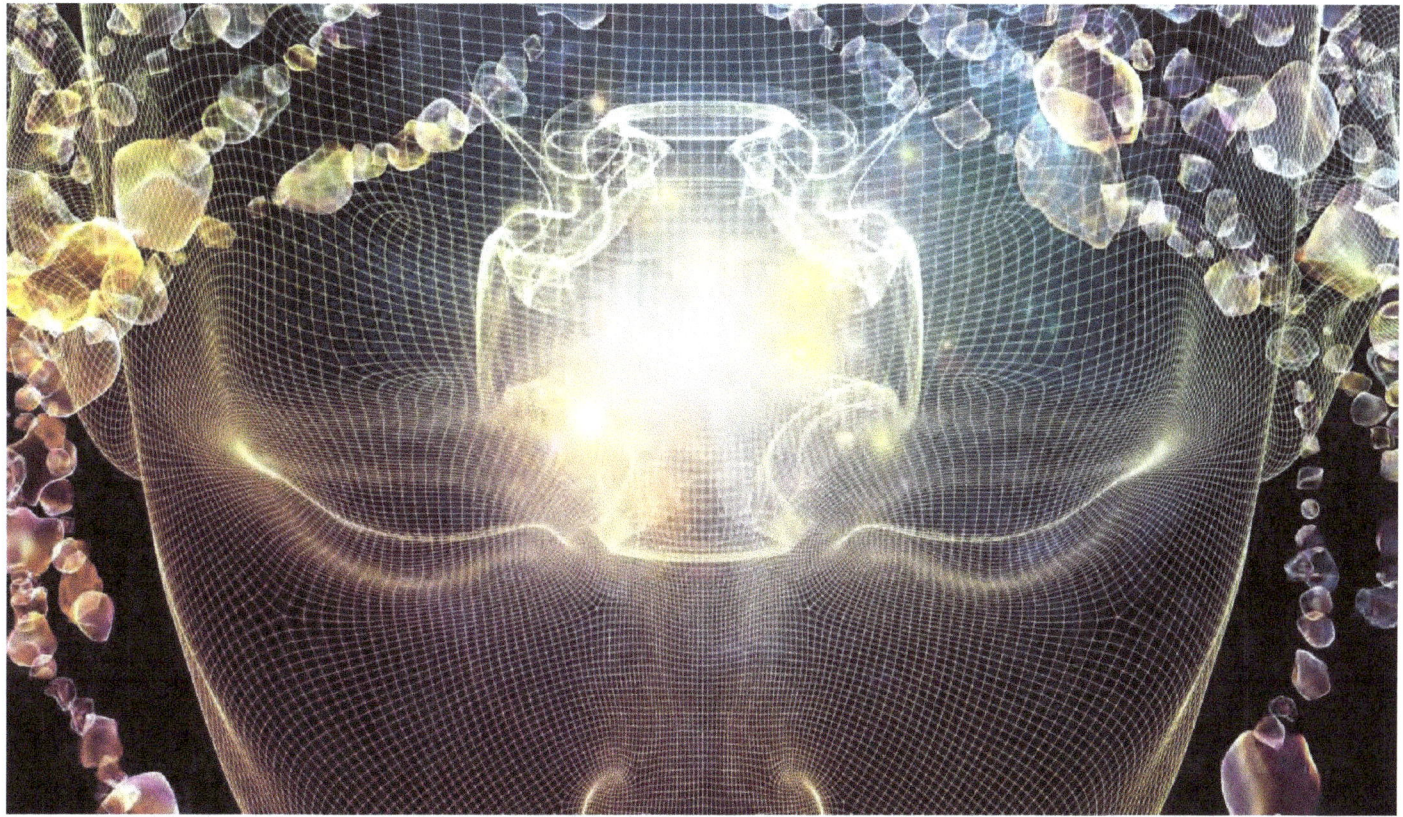

8. The teacher and helper's (therapist's) role is just that: helping the individual achieve clarity, accept responsibility and learn the proper method to access their soul. Like a gardener, who tears out the weeds allowing the flowers to emerge.

9. Two major obstacles in this process are:
a) **Denial.** The inability to recognize the existence of a problem, which of course compounds the problem many times over and has a snowball effect of adding on layer after layer of new distortions and complications. Half the cure is awareness of the illness.
b) **Confusion** caused by the mix of healthy and unhealthy behavior mechanisms. This makes it extremely difficult to distinguish between the two, which in turn adds to the denial process.

10. The basic necessary requirements of a good teacher and therapist:
a) **Care and sensitivity.**

b) Empathy.
c) Wisdom.
d) Knowledge and experience, competence and skill, in the study of human nature.
e) Trusting.
f) Humility.
g) **Absolute respect for human dignity and independence;** that every person has to assume personal responsibility for his behavior. In Jewish terms: Complete faith in God and the divine soul in each person created in God's own image.
h) **Total conviction** that all human experiences are part of a process of growth.
i) **Flexibility and imagination**. Appreciating and respecting the differences between people and thus not fit them in to any mold (while not compromising #h).
j) Recognition of one's own limitations and subjectivity.
k) Methodology and technique.
l) **Acceptance without question** of all the above requirements.

The process of therapy generally breaks down into the following steps:
1. Establishing trust and opening a channel of communication.

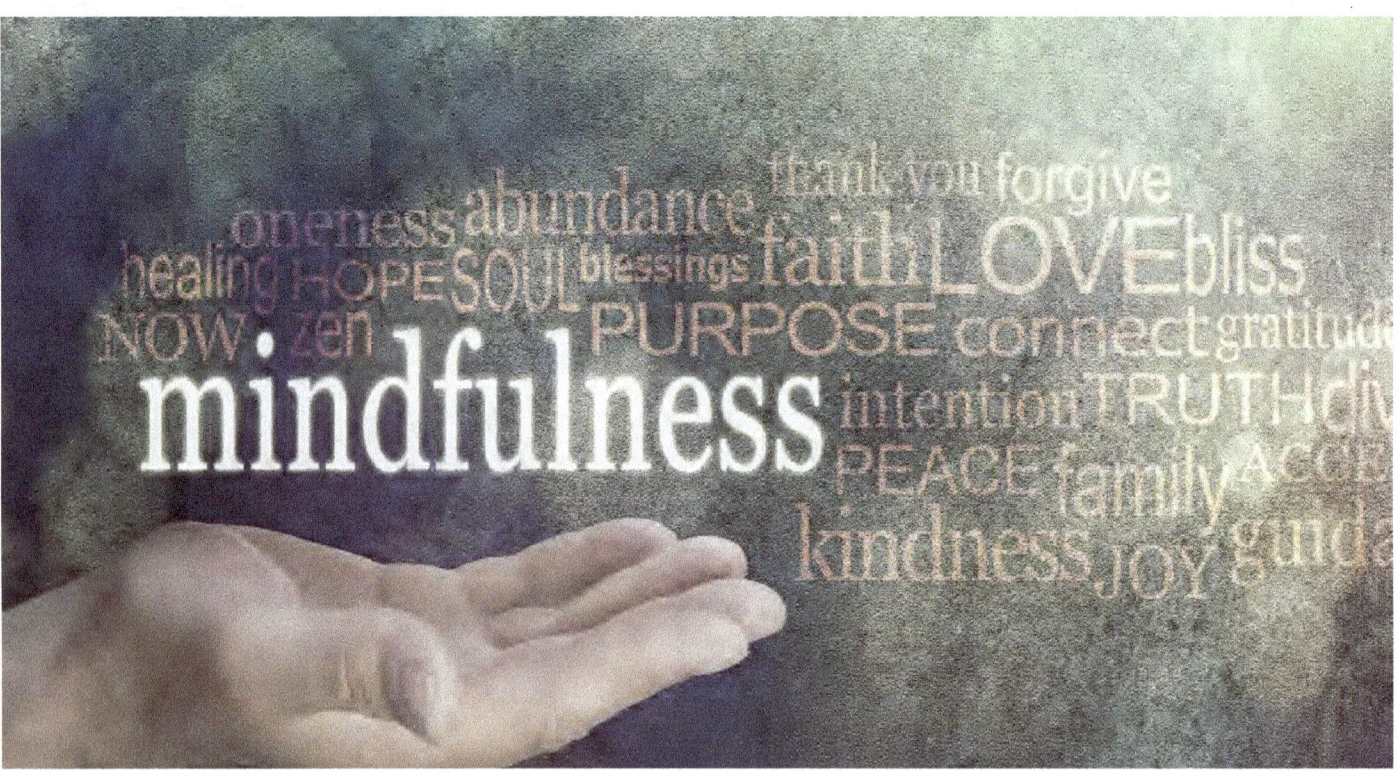

2. Hearing the problems and helping define them from the student or client's perspective.

3. Guiding the client to slowly redefine the problems from a more honest and objective perspective. Including an examination of the client's responses and blind-spots.

4. Establishing that the client is responsible for himself [if he is not, than he needs another form of help]. Defining what that responsibility entails.

5. Specifying and defining unequivocally the roles of therapist and client. Making it absolutely clear that the therapist is trained only to help the client help himself. The therapist provides care and support, but is not a crutch and does not initiate the cry and need for help. It is not a personal, reciprocal relationship. These points have to be emphasized time and again, as deemed necessary.

6. Recognizing if this particular therapist-client dynamic is not going to work. This can be for a variety of reasons, including sometimes the humble recognition on the part of the therapist that the best therapist can only help one who is willing to help himself, which often needs the client to have hit rock-bottom and desperately seek help. No therapist can replace that cry for help.

7. Developing a process of movement and growth with the intended goal to rise up above yourself and relate to a higher reality. This must be done in a step by step basis, timed at the pace of the client, enabling him to internalize it.

8. Defining the objective in simple terms. Consistently reviewing the goal and illustrating how all the many elaborate steps in reaching the goal are but a means to that higher end. Establishing this is crucial in the process, firstly because it gives the client (and the therapist) a sense of direction and keeps him from wandering off due to different distractions. Second, it treats the client with respect, knowing that he is being guided to help himself, and empowers the client with the feeling of control over his own life.

9. Persistence and tenacity, never losing sight of the initial goal.

10. Consistency in the devotion and care for the client.

11. Assurance and reassurance of progress. Acknowledging the potential and, indeed, need for setbacks; but recognizing that the primary goal is not how quick and how far one reaches, but steady movement rather than inertia. Emphasizing that any movement, frontwards or backwards, any sensation, pain or pleasure, anger or joy, is better than lethargy and numbness.

12. Frequent review (with an objective party) of the therapist's decision-making process. With special emphasis on the therapist's attitudes and feelings.

13. Recognizing when to let go. When to allow the client to walk (or fly) on his own, even at the expense of falling. Only then can he truly learn to walk on his own. Actually this should be rephrased: During the entire therapeutic process the client should be walking (and falling) on his own with gentle guidance from the therapist. The therapist must recognize if the client is becoming to dependent on the therapist and then help him become self-dependent.

Pitfalls to be wary of from the client's side:
1. An overly manipulative client who wants to engage the therapist in battle or enjoys mind-games.
Solution: If the therapist is unable to make any progress due to the client's attitude – confront (sometimes gently) the client. Establish the reasons for his attitude and if it can be overcome. If not – make it clear to the client why the therapy cannot continue under such circumstances.

2. Overdependence on the therapist. This is a particularly sticky problem because:
a) the client needs to trust the therapist and often has trust issues with a pattern of no one to depend on in life,
b) of the frequent need for "transference."
Solution: Absolute faith and respect of an individual's personal space and responsibility, recognizing that no one (even with the greatest effort) can ever enter into the "alone" space (the most intimate space) of another individual. That is how God created humans. In the words of Hillel: "Im ayn Ani Le Mi Le," "If I am not for myself who will be for me." The trained and G-d- fearing therapist knows that "Im ani l'atzmi moh ani," "If I am for myself what am I," doesn't compromise the "I", but only comes to teach us that with the help of another one can learn to enhance and access their own "I". Only with absolute acceptance of G-d can a human therapist learn to rise above himself and help another with total devotion, and give the client confidence that his dependence on the therapist will not compromise the client's "I". (see also below)

Pitfalls to be wary of from the therapist's side:
3. An overly manipulative therapist. Especially an intelligent one who can manipulate the client, even if it's in the client's

> **The therapist must recognize if the client is becoming to dependent on the therapist and then help him become self-dependent.**

best interest. Where do you draw the line between healthy and unhealthy manipulation?

4. The sense of control that a therapist assumes over the client's life hearing the client's most intimate issues, without any reciprocity.

5. The affirmation a therapist gets from the client's trust in him which can lead to a reverse dependence or "counter-transference."

Solution (to #3-5 above): In addition to the obvious methods of constant case review particularly with an objective supervisor, the Torah requires of the therapist an uncompromising selflessness, total egolessness, to the extreme that the therapist has to be the harshest judge of himself, and he must subject himself to total scrutiny by someone he respects and trusts.

The therapist's approach in dealing with a client must be with the greatest awe and humility, recognizing the enormous responsibility he carries of being allowed to enter into the most sacred, intimate recesses of the soul of G-d's child. He has to visualize G-d standing over him at all times and watching carefully: how are you dealing with my child? Nothing less is required of the therapist.

Finding Oneness In **Diversity**

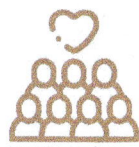

Something that strikes us (even subjectively) as beautiful is balance and symmetry of several – or very many – different elements, all combined in just the right blend.

One of the great challenges and ostensible paradoxes is reconciling between the individual and the collective, between personal interests and the common good. Can we find a way to preserve our diversity while being united without either being compromised?

The way to achieve this balance is through humility: When you sublimate yourself to a higher calling, your individuality unites, instead of separates you with others serving the greater cause. Your powerful commitment permeates your being to the point that it tempers self-interest, not allowing it to rip you apart from others. On the contrary, it helps build a unified community – diverse but united by a cause greater than, and one that transcends, individual interests. Yet, it takes effort on your part as an individual to find this harmony in diversity. Here is why the effort is worth it.

Beauty In Diversity

As pretty as one color – say, blue – may be, it still would not be defined as beautiful. As sweet as one musical note may sound, it cannot be called beautiful. Beauty is always a combination of many colors – as in a painting – whose

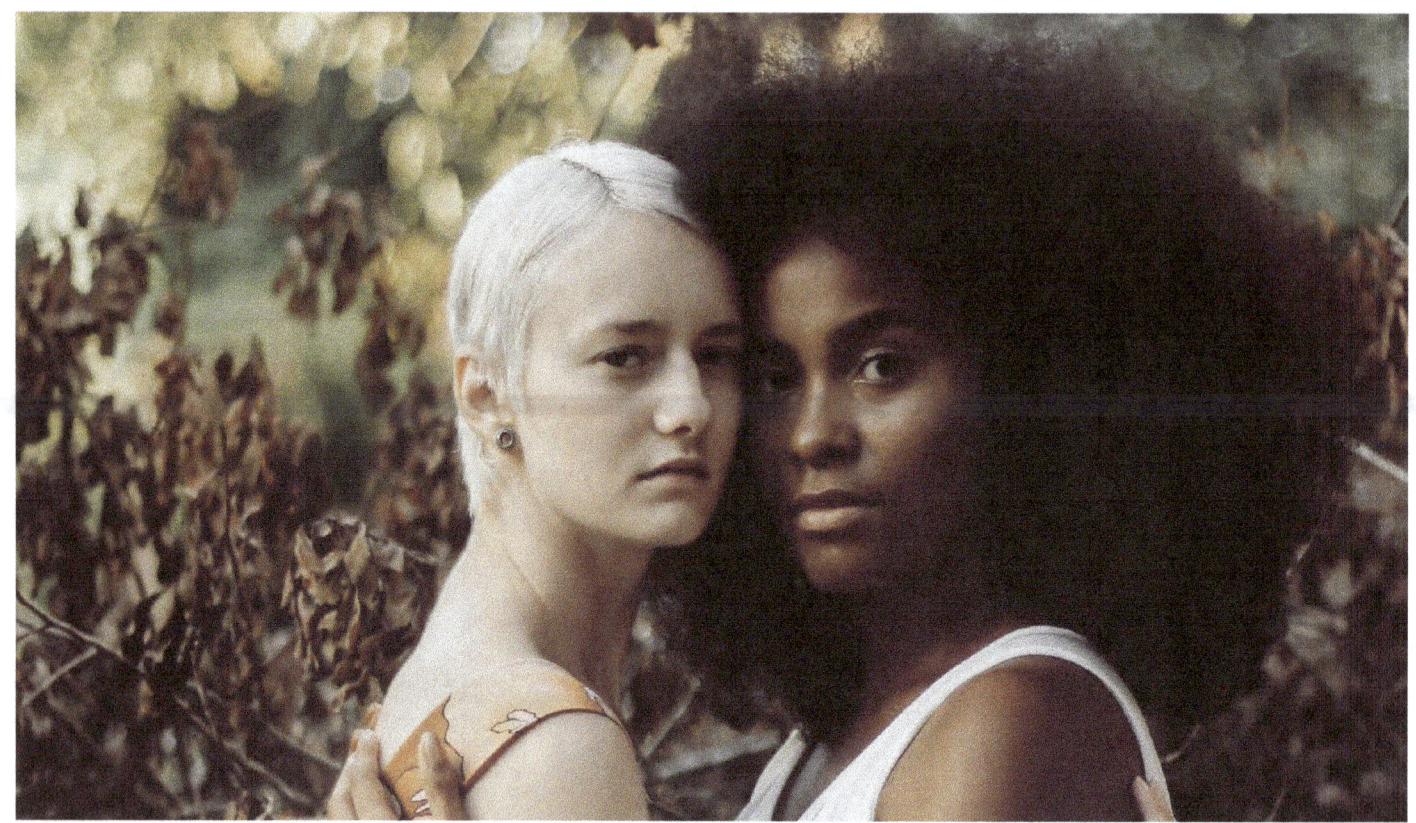

balance and coordination creates a beautiful mosaic. Many different musical notes, when played just the right way, generate a beautiful symphony.

Take nature.
The beauty of nature is in the fact that so many different systems work together with such astonishing synchronicity. Perhaps no better or closer example of this is our own selves. The healthy human body is a miraculous piece of architecture. So many different limbs and organs, numerous diverse systems and faculties. Let alone the multitude of cells, hormones, chemicals, and DNA. And all combined as one fascinating unit, working as one synchronized whole. Something that strikes us (even subjectively) as beautiful is balance and symmetry of several – or very many – different elements, all combined in just the right blend.

Beauty: the harmony within diversity.
Humility in Diversity
We are all one: Together we comprise a single organism whose

various cells, limbs, and organs complement and complete one another. A body includes both the sophisticated, refined brain and the "crass" functional foot; but, ultimately, the brain is dependent on the foot just as the foot is dependent on the brain. If the foot is indebted to the brain for its vitality and direction, the brain is dependent on the foot to realize many of its goals.

The humble man looks at the larger picture rather than the particulars, at the unified purpose of life on earth rather than only at his function within this purpose. No matter how lofty his own role may seem in relation to his fellow's, he is grossly limited without him. The knowledge that his own life's work is incomplete without his fellow's contribution arouse feelings of humility and indebtedness toward his fellow: He recognizes that every "limb" of the mutual body is indispensable, every component complements and advances his interest.

Defining Humility

In this approach, humility is not equated with a sense of inferiority. Rather, it stems from a feeling of equality and mutual need. In becoming humble, you first realize not to feel superior about your unique qualities and strengths: All the virtues you have been blessed with — whether it is a greater measure of intelligence, refinement, or spiritual sensitivity — are only the tools that have been granted you to fulfill your mission in life. You recognize that your own accomplishments require the collaboration with others. Be humbled by the fact that every single individual on earth has a unique and irreplaceable role to play, and that every one is both needed and needs all the others.

"

Be humbled by the fact that every single individual on earth has a unique and irreplaceable role to play, and that every one is both needed and needs all the others.

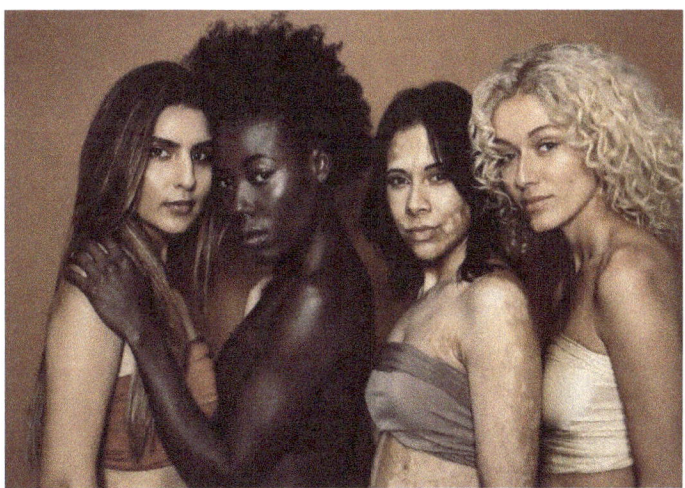

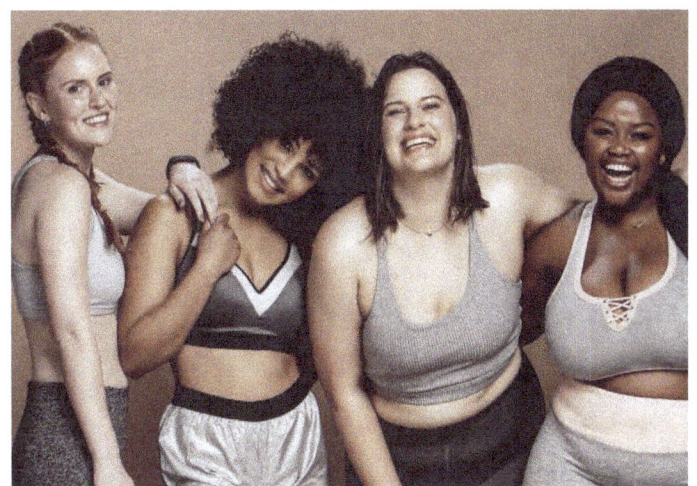

Mindfulness

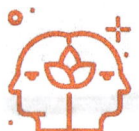

It is critical that we believe in ourselves to be able to achieve anything in this world. That we can touch the infinite and the eternal.

How to Make Your Actions Matter

Do you feel burned out? Jaded? Like nothing matters anymore? Like the problems of the world are so endemic and entrenched that you can't even make a small dent in them? There is one key to making your actions matter — faith. Not a juvenile or simple faith — but a confidence in the higher unknown that lies beyond the rational. If you can expand your world to include what you cannot explain or understand, you're on the way to making your actions matter. How? Read on.

A Platform for a Life of Meaning and Purpose

True and healthy faith creates a platform for a life of meaning and purpose, a life in which our actions matter and our experiences are driven with direction. While a life of no belief may feel alright, it renders life as a random set of circumstances, with survival of the fittest being the cardinal rule. We live in a world in which we are being taught that people are essentially selfish creatures, driven by self-interest. In the Darwinian-Freudian model of life, which is the prevalent theory impacting every aspect of our existence, our psyches are being continuously inundated with how insignificant our lives truly are. The driving ethos of all creatures as "natural selection" basically renders every human virtue, every noble act, every thing we hold dear, as a method for billion-year-old bacteria to adapt and survive.

The Soul Is Beyond Selfishness

While its true that every person has a selfish inclination, we also have a transcendent side, which is capable of the noblest behavior. The deepest part of the human being is the soul rather than the "id." The essence of the soul is a bulletproof, eternal source of goodness. The easier route may be the narcissistic one. But the more meaningful route is the benevolent one. A person always has the choice to overcome his/her primitive temptations and access the transcendent soul within. The soul is a rich resource, with layers and layers of potential. The challenge is to recognize and draw forth this dimension, which can lay concealed beneath the outer shell of material survival.

Believe in Yourself

"Impossible. Absolutely impossible." How often do we hear these discouraging words, pouring cold water on our freshly hatched ideas? Don't you think that the first inventors of the airplane or any other technology were told by their peers that their dreams were an impossibility? Yet, they persisted and finally prevailed. History is witness to countless stories of humans achieving the impossible.

And how else do we explain the seemingly irrational — or more accurately: supra-rational — drive that we can overcome any challenge. How, for instance, are doctors utterly convinced that they can ultimately conquer every illness?! It is because we have an instinct that all is possible. This instinct stems from the power of the soul — the inherent faith and trust we carry in our soul — that transcends mortality and all the limits and shortcomings of human existence.

It is critical that we believe in ourselves to be able to achieve anything in this world. That we can touch the infinite and the eternal. But we must also know that our psyches are under a constant assault of many forces reminding us time and again about our limitations, feeding our insecurities and fears. You have the power to be Divine, and with ease! You only need to believe that it is possible.

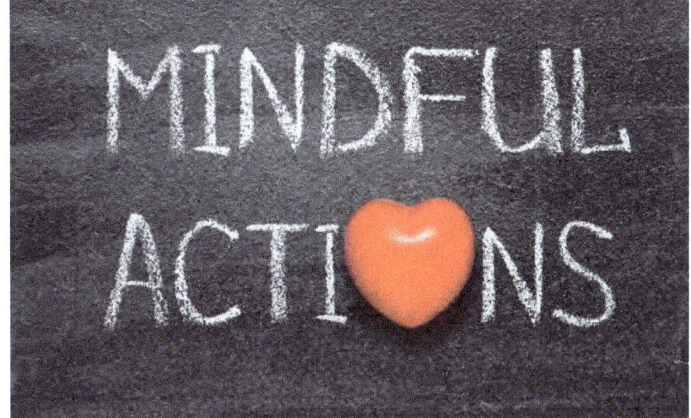

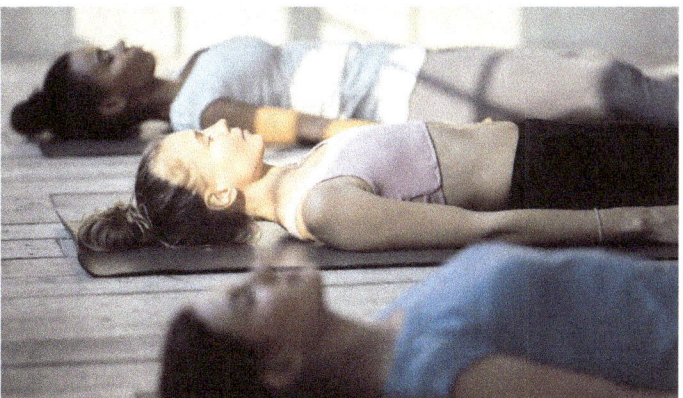

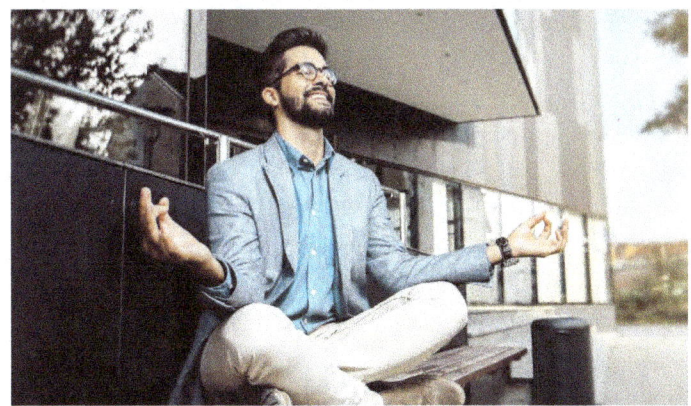

Individuality in Judaism

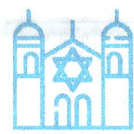

Judaism is considered by religious Jews to be the expression of the covenant that God established with the Children of Israel.

There are two paths of Judaism and Mysticism

Judaism
Judaism is an ethnic religion comprising the collective religious, cultural and legal tradition and civilization of the Jewish people. Judaism is considered by religious Jews to be the expression of the covenant that God established with the Children of Israel. It encompasses a wide body of texts, practices, theological positions, and forms of organization. They include the following groups.

Conservative
Conservative Judaism is a kind of middle ground between Reform and Modern Orthodox. The name comes from the idea of trying to "conserve" traditions rather than leaving them unchanged or full-out reforming them. Services are often a mix of Hebrew and English and there may be male and female rabbis, cantors, and educators. There's a wide range of observance among Conservative Jews: Some keep kosher, some don't; some refrain from work and driving on Shabbat, some don't. In the 1970s, it was the biggest movement in American Judaism. It's gotten smaller over time as more people have chosen to go toward one of the other multitudes of choices — or nothing, which is that part that makes us sad.

Being conservative has nothing to do with who you vote for (except maybe for Sisterhood president). Culturally Jewish/Jewish-ish/

JewCurious
These are the people who have a Jewish heritage but aren't really into it or

connected in any meaningful way. They probably identify more with bagels and Seinfeld than with prayers or synagogues. Their Jewish identity might come from going to an annual Passover Seder, celebrating the High Holidays, having had a bris (yeah, that's a daily reminder), or fond memories of their Bar/Bat Mitzvah party. Or maybe it's just the thought of their grandmother's latkes. They may sometimes want to connect with the religious part, like when a relative dies and it's time to sit shiva, but it's not an everyday thing.

There are lots of reasons people feel more Jewish-ish than Jewish, like having one Jewish parent, or a non-Jewish partner, or not having observed any Jewish ritual growing up. The thing about this group is that it is likely a single-generation phenomenon. The Judaism seems to weaken with every generation. A typical example of this is that in 1945, the grandparents kept kosher and joined a synagogue. In 1969, the parents just joined a synagogue. In 1998, the kid just felt culturally Jewish and in 2020, what then? On the other hand, folks who are Jew-Curious may or may not have Jewish heritage, but they do have some interest in learning about Judaism. Someone who married into a Jewish family, or maybe just someone who wants to learn more about the religion, because who wouldn't, might be considered JewCurious.

If you're JewCurious, you've come to the right place, 'cause you've got questions, and we've got answers!

Disengaged Jews (DJs)

Our target market... come to Mama!

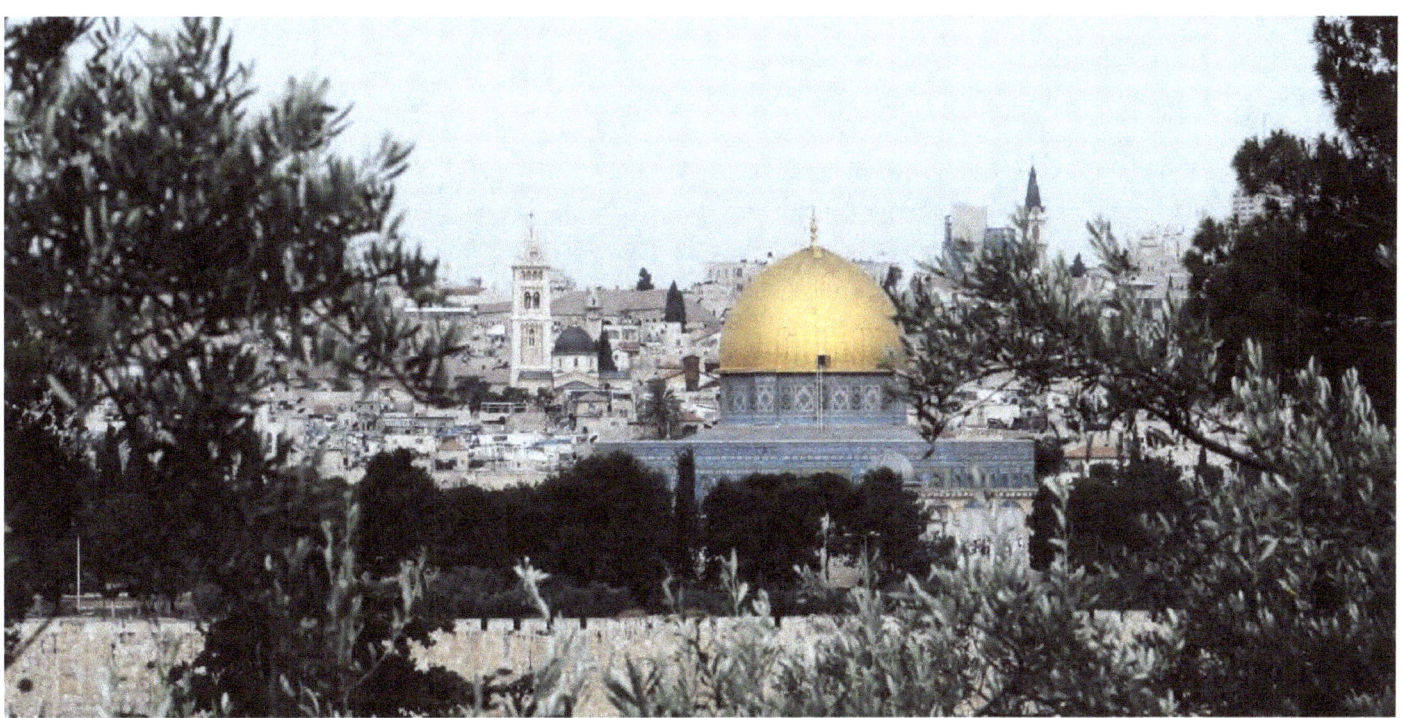

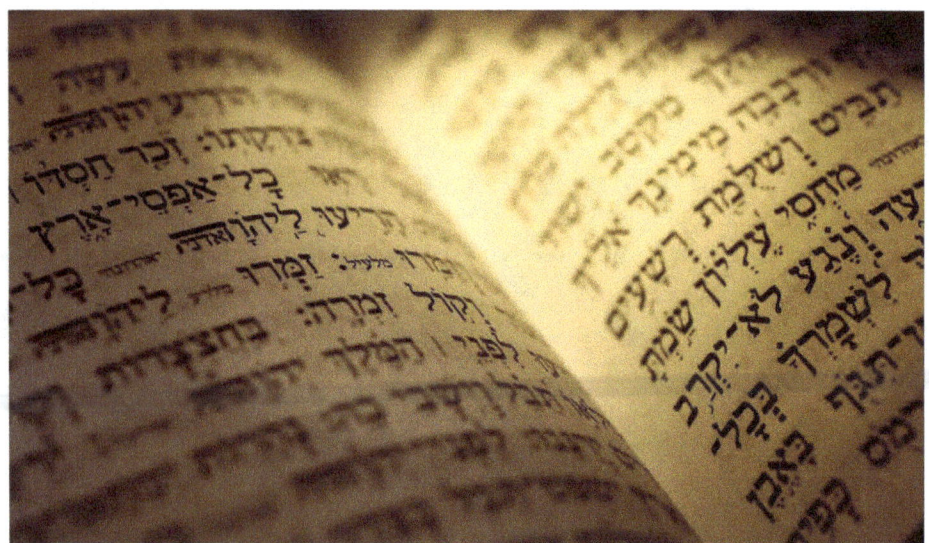

Disengaged Jews are arguably the biggest group of Jews and they are doing very little, if anything, Jewish — yet. Sometimes with Judaism it's easy to feel like you don't belong. We sooo get it. That's literally why our name and tagline is JewBelong: for when you feel you don't! This is the group that JewBelong was created for. And if you're not a DJ, please think about the DJs in your life and consider sharing JewBelong with them.

Modern Orthodox

Modern Orthodox Jews generally follow religious law strictly, but they are also full participants in modern society. They generally keep kosher, observe Shabbat with an all-the-rules approach, belong to a synagogue and go to services, have children in Jewish day school, and so on. Most Modern Orthodox men wear kippot or yarmulkes. (Actually, most Modern Orthodox men wear those crocheted yarmulkes.) Modern Orthodox women run the gamut from those who cover their hair with a pretty scarf, or some who might wear a wig in public. Or some who don't cover their hair at all, except probably in synagogue. And no halter tops or booty shorts for Modern Orthodox women — they dress modestly with shirts that cover their shoulders and skirts that go to the knee. You can't always tell if someone is Modern Orthodox just by the way they dress.

Non-denominational, Post-denominational, Unaffiliated

Well, duh, of course, look at the joke at the beginning of this section. What with all the Jewish movements, there just has to be room for all of those folks who just don't fit into any of them. At this point, these affiliations are more of an art than a science and you gotta feel for these poor rabbis who are simply trying to lead a community of Jews whose taste and interests are constantly changing. TBH, if you take a look in the larger Jewish cities, like New York, L.A., or Chicago, there are some very cool unaffiliated synagogues worth checking out.
The biggest group of Jews are the Disengaged Jews, or DJs for short (although you may or may not want them picking the tunes at your next pool party).

Reconstructionist

Reconstructionist Judaism lands somewhere between Conservative and Reform. It started as an offshoot of the Conservative movement but today it's closer to Reform. Services and observance seem traditional, but the overarching idea is that Jewish values and practices take precedence over religious rules and traditions. Reconstructionist Judaism seems to work well for interfaith families or Jews by choice. It's heavier on meaning, welcoming and spirituality than on dogma.

Reconstructionism sometimes seems a little hippy-ish or granola but we kind of love that!

Reform

The Reform movement is known for being less bound to rule-following and more focused on Jewish values. Maybe not coincidentally, it's the largest group of North American Jews. Progressive, inclusive, and committed to equal rights (even before being all those things was a thing), it was the first organized movement to ordain women as rabbis and cantors and to elect women as presidents of synagogues. Reform services are often in English (sometimes with a guitar or other musical instrument), and people often don't wear yarmulkes or tallit. If you listen closely, you can sometimes hear more observant Jews bitch about the Reform Movement saying it's barely Jewish or Jewish lite, and they are not saying it like it's a compliment. That being said, plenty of people, including us, love the Reform movement.

Want to go to services that are mostly in English? The Reform movement might be for you!

Secular

Yup, you can be an atheist and a Jew. One of the coolest things about Judaism is that it does not demand belief in God to be a good Jew. It puts acts

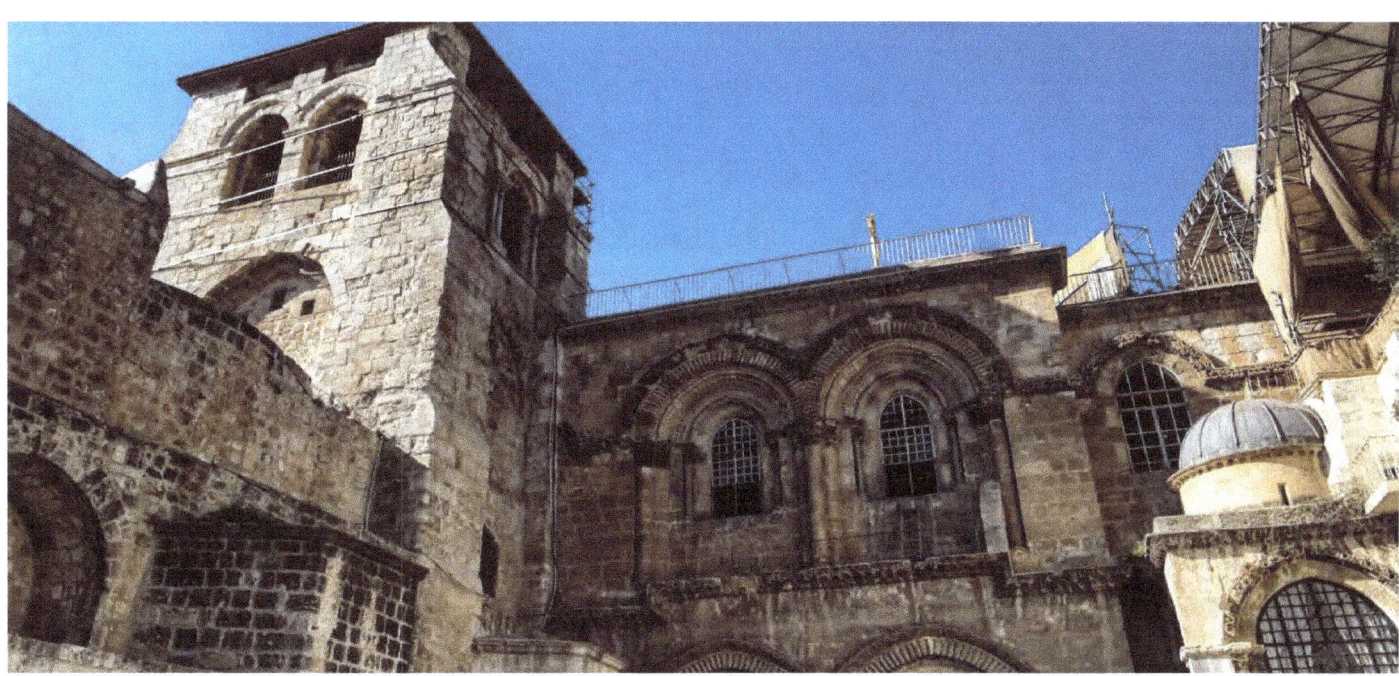

of kindness in front of faith. Secular Jews often include Jewish traditions and values in their lives. Some may also belong to a synagogue or another Jewish community that does Jewish stuff but that don't have a big focus on the God parts. Almost half of American Jews consider themselves Secular or somewhat Secular, according to a Pew study that was done in 2013. So yeah, this is a big group.

Yup, we're gonna say it. You don't need to believe in God to be a "good Jew." (Seriously though, the term "good Jew" kind of gives us hives.)

Ultra-Orthodox

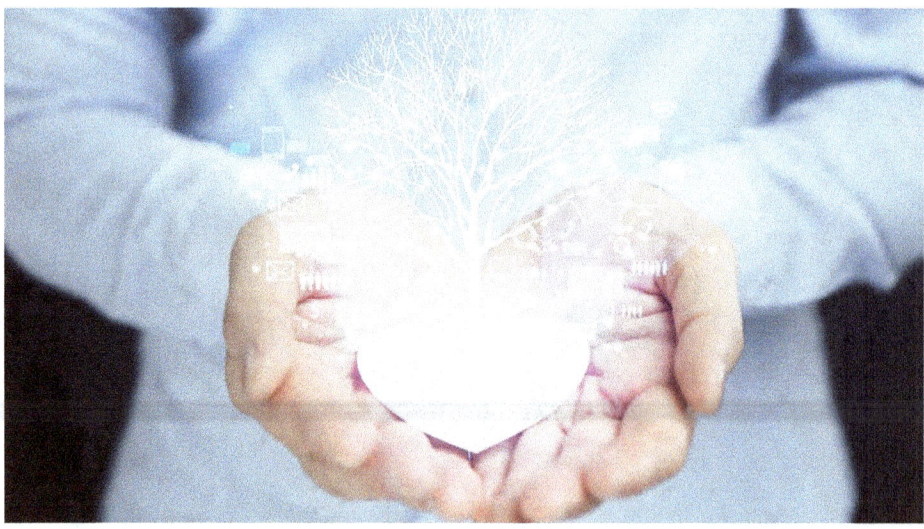

Also known as Haredi or Hasidic Jews, these are the folks you see wearing black coats and hats with beards and, depending on their tradition, payot (side curls). Women are generally covered head to toe as well, and many wear wigs to cover their hair once they are married. (And no, according to the Ultra-Orthodox Jews we've asked, they don't mind the heat any more than most do.) Men and women sit separately in Ultra-Orthodox synagogues, and women aren't allowed to participate in some of the rituals, like reading from the Torah. It's a broad group of people with many separate communities, but the one thing they generally agree on is that modern secular culture is not for them. Ultra-Orthodox communities tend to be tight-knit and focused around religious practice and guidelines. There's also a group called the Jewish Renewal movement, which, according to their website "combines the ecstatic prayer of Hasidic Judaism with a contemporary ethos of gender egalitarianism, environmental consciousness, progressive politics and appreciation of religious diversity," which sounds nice, but it's a pretty small group. Paradoxically, Chabad is an Ultra-Orthodox organization, but their focus is on Jewish outreach and they go out of their way to be welcoming, especially toward those with less knowledge of Jewish tradition.

Mysticism

Academic study of Jewish mysticism, especially since Gershom Scholem's Major Trends in Jewish Mysticism (1941), distinguishes between different forms of mysticism across different eras of Jewish history. Of these, Kabbalah, which emerged in 12th-century Europe, is the most well known, but not the only typologic form, or the earliest to emerge. Among previous forms were Merkabah mysticism (c. 100 BC – 1000 AD), and Ashkenazi Hasidim (early 13th century AD) around the time of Kabbalistic emergence and Messianic Judaism.

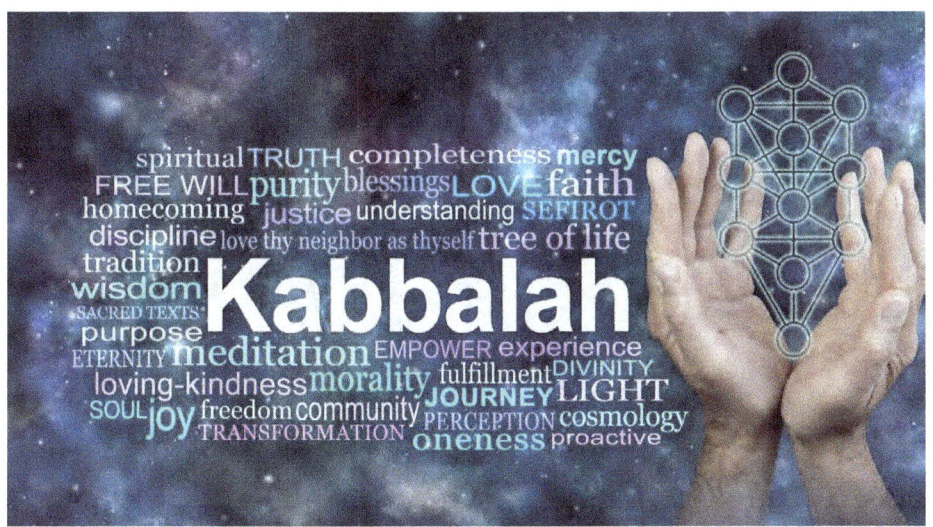

Individuality in Judaism

Indeed, in my opinion, the question of individuality in Judaism is one of the most important ones in our times, and addresses one of today's greatest distortions – and is root of a profound stereotype – which has become the source of endless anxiety and divisiveness.

How often lately has the debate cropped up between religious advocates ardently dictating certain standards and equally passionate positions advocating personal freedoms? Whether it is abortion, the right to die or other expressions of choice, it seems like an irresolvable dispute.

How many people have turned away from their heritage because they felt their souls were asphyxiated by the demands of religious conformity (I use the word "asphyxiated" intentionally – read on why).

The dilemma is obvious: Religion dictates the rigid commitment to an absolute system of laws and guidelines; individuality is the free expression of your unique personality, independent of any system's orders. Religion demands conformity; conformity is the antithesis of individuality.

This at least is the perception of most people, including many who have embraced a religious lifestyle.

Some argue that the justification for suppressing individuality in the name of religion is that left on our own, people can gravitate to anarchy. The benefits of religious discipline outweigh the virtues of independent expression, and therefore justify its suppression. However the major flaw in this argument is that faith dictates that the same G-d that gave humans guidelines also created them as individuals, each with their own unique personalities, mindsets and dispositions. "Their faces are not alike, their minds are not alike."

From the beginning of time no two people ever existed that are alike! Indeed, the Mishne states: "Why was the human created as an individual? To teach us [our great individual responsibility] that each person must say 'the entire universe was created for me.'"

Yes, some obstinate religionists may argue that our inherent individuality can be seen as the "enemy," no different than the "evil inclination." According to this thinking, G-d gave us individuality as a challenging voice that must be suppressed, lest we risk undermining the "system." I don't believe we need to spend time refuting this argument.

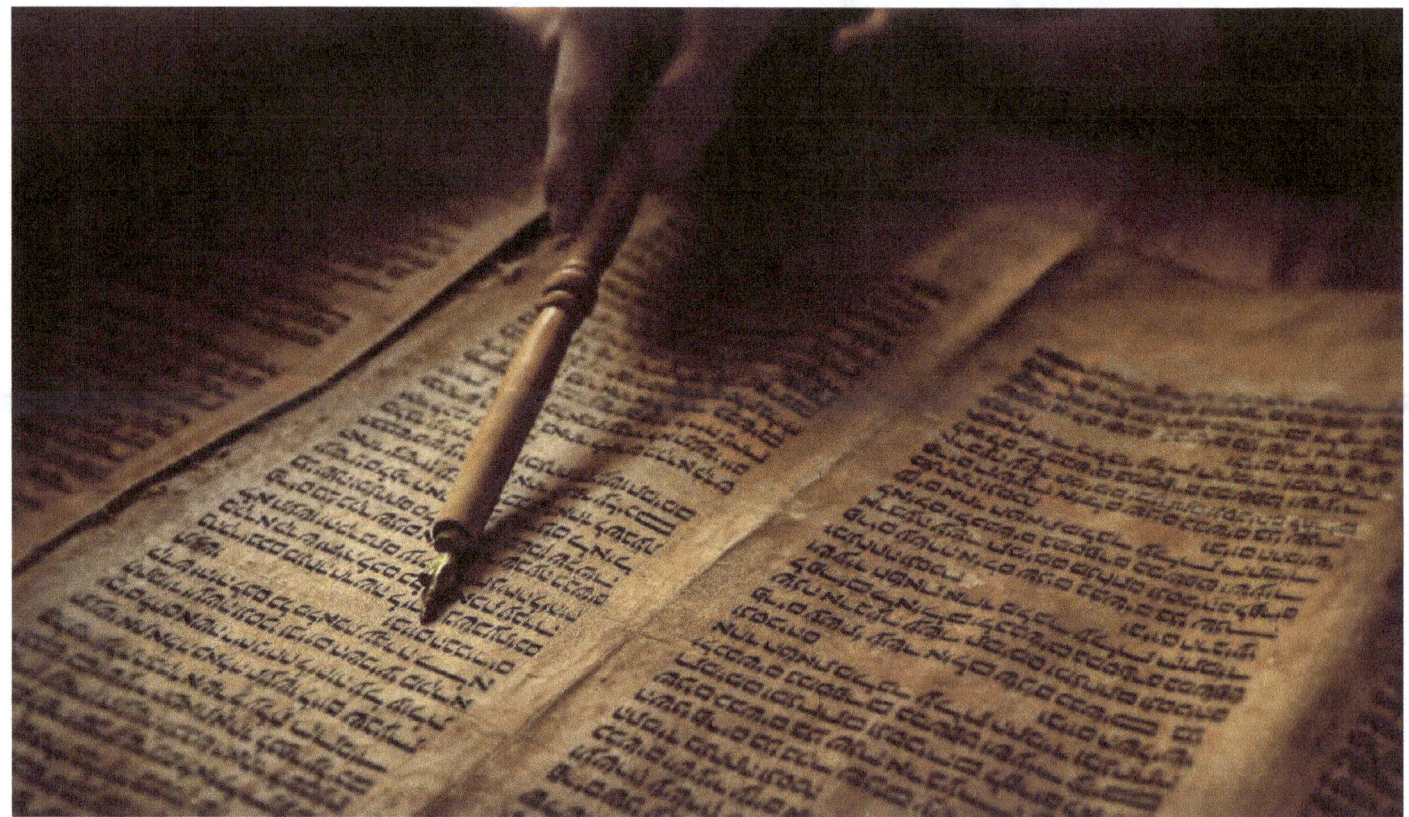

Suffice it to say that according to this "thinking" no single innovation, no unique contribution, no unique melody would ever have been played in history had people suppressed their individuality in the name of religious conformity! Can we really say that G-d created so many different people just in order that they all shed their differences and become self-made clones?! Is such a thing even possible...

So how do we reconcile our individuality with the seemingly inflexible discipline of religion? Whenever addressing any given issue, especially one shrouded in controversy as well as touching a deep personal place, it is critical to first dispel myths and distortions that cloud the essential issue. Then we can look at the issue itself with new eyes and perhaps discover its original intent.

When discussing religion we must distinguish between man-made established systems that may or may not reflect on the true meaning of faith, and the true meaning of faith.

I submit that most (if not all) opposition to religious ideas is based on the way people and their institutions have projected these ideas.

For me "I feel deeply Jewish. And I was hungering for some answers, for some spiritual nourishment. Instead I was being invalidated and silenced. I was dying inside. I was just not made to be a conformist. I attended Messianic Church most of my life which is considered a form of Mysticism to most Jews.

"I found my answer in Mysticism. I found the Seven heavens of Christ. With each level my personal identity and purpose is developed.

After all I did not reject school because I understood that in school we are on an individual journey even though we are all learning the same information. I am challenged to always question and seek questions that will bring me further to purpose, identity and untimely oneness with G-d.

In the beginning I am

○ First heaven
The Seed of Faith and acceptance in the "oneness" of the Tree of Life design

○ Second heaven
I am reborn: Within me are 2 paths: one that will lead me to the tree of life and one that will lead me to the tree of Good and Evil.

○ Third heaven
My destiny must and transportation to the next level must be decided.

○ Forth heaven
Understanding how to use power for purpose is key in the fourth level

○ Fifth heaven
I begin my journey to purging all ungodly motives

○ Sixth heaven
Wisdom is being a leader that can teach the teachers truth.

○ Seventh heaven
I am a part of the Tree of Life; a mediator between mankind and God.

I shared with her the following analogy: When the nightingale was created with a beautiful voice, she came complaining to G-d: "I thank you for my beautiful voice. I love to sing into the night. However my voice also attracts predators. A hungry animal looking for a nice meal will be drawn to my voice. Seeing a piece of flesh, a little bird, perched on a branch, they will pursue me for their next meal. Please G-d, give me a defense with which I can protect myself from predators."

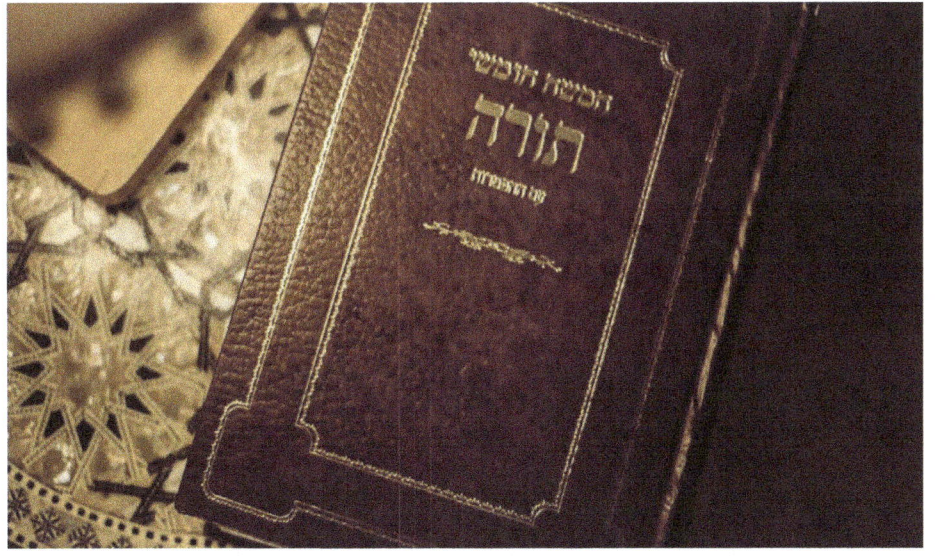

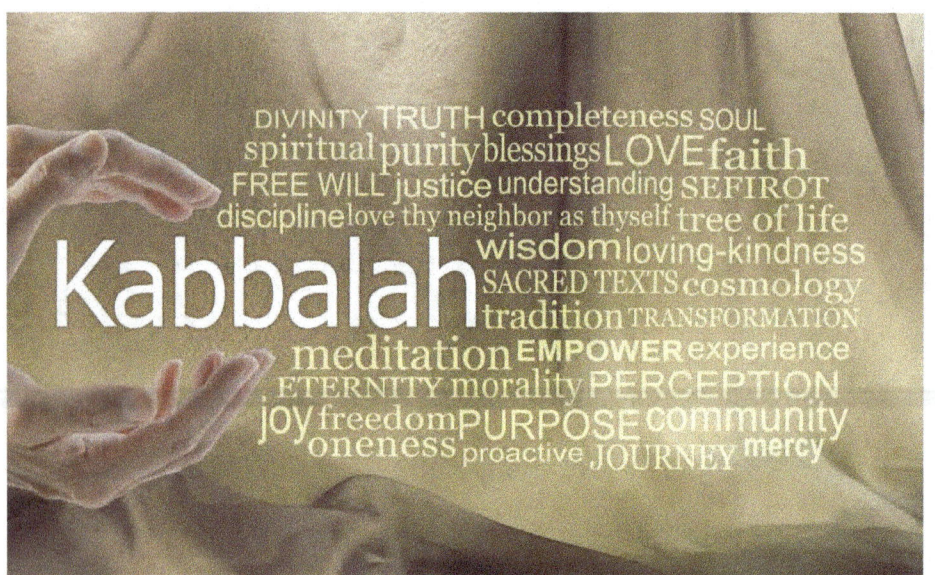

G-d offered the bird a beak. The nightingale examined the merchandise and declined it, saying: "Please G-d. I'm a beautiful bird. A nose like that is unbecoming for an elegant bird like me." G-d then offered the bird claws. And again, the bird rejected them: "Such ugly long nails – so unbecoming." Finally G-d offered the bird a set of wings. The bird looked at the two wings and exclaimed: "Master of the Universe. You created us all with profound wisdom and design. I don't understand. I have enough body weight to carry with me when I need to escape predators. You're now giving me two more pieces of flesh that just add more weight and will make it more difficult for me to escape!"

G-d replied: "No, little bird. Let me tell you. I'll teach you how to use these wings. I will teach you to soar. With these wings you'll be able to fly away and escape your enemies."

Mitzvot – the laws of the Torah – are commitments that clearly add more "body weight" and responsibility to a person's life. It's easier and lighter to live a life without responsibility. Yet, if you only see the "body" of the mitzvot then they can appear as "dead weight." However when you learn to access their soul, you discover their ability to serve as "wings" to fly with; wings that lift and carry you to places you could never reach on you own.

There is no bird in the world (even one wanting to lose weight…) that would prefer to be wingless. It's sad to see a grounded bird that cannot fly. What's even sadder, I told the woman, is a bird that has wings and doesn't know that it does or how to use them.

Unfortunately, an oppressive home and a dogmatic education can clip our wings, or conceal the fact that we have them. In place we are left with a lot of body weight.

Mitzvot mean not merely commandments (that's their "body" translation). They mean connections – they are wings that connect us to our own essence, to our calling, to our destiny.

And therein lies the eloquent integration of religious discipline and individuality: If mitzvot were superimposed guidelines, then they would contradict our unique personalities, and the only way to embrace them would be to conform and suppress our individual selves. However, as connections mitzvot actually uncover the true inherent nature of the human being. They are wings that allow our souls to soar to the greatest heights. A good example for this is the discipline of music. Anyone who wishes to play or compose music must "conform" to this absolute, immutable system. But this not called "conforming; it's called "freeing." By submitting to this framework, the musician will be able to uncover the true power of music and create a melody that touches the deepest place in a person's heart, and transports us to unprecedented heights. Imagine, then, a musical discipline whose laws are dictated by the inventor and creator of life—by the one who has intimate knowledge of life's every strength and every vulnerability, of its every potential and its every sensitivity.

Yes, the Torah offers us spiritual paragons and ethical models for us to live up to; we are taught to emulate Abraham, Isaac and Jacob, and Sarah, Rivkah, Rachel and Leah. But not in order to squash our personalities and unique talents; on the contrary: to be inspired by these great people to use our individuality to express our deepest faculties.

> Mitzvot mean not merely commandments (that's their "body" translation). **They mean connections – they are wings that connect us to our own essence, to our calling, to our destiny.**

The big myth is that Judaism is about conformity. The earliest roots of Judaism all about rebellion against the status quo. The first Jew – and father of all nations – was the first revolutionary: he shattered the idols in his father's home and rebelled against the entire standard of living of his times. Abraham instilled that revolutionary spirit into his children. Coming from Purim, Mordechai would not bow to Haman. Throughout history people of true faith stood out with their revolutionary attitude – refusing to conform to the norm of the land, and setting a visionary course to a brighter future.

I believe that the reason so many religious institutions gravitate toward suppression rather than encourage the unique voice is out of fear and insecurity. It seems easier to keep people in line by suppressing individual expression; many are more aware of the body of Torah than its soul. When we lack the confidence in the soul's ability to soar, we often tend to put on "blinders" and retreat toward the comfort of conformity.

Our education system must be revived with the spirit of faith: To teach our children how traditional disciplines are musical notes; how they are wings that allow us to fly and express our deepest selves.

Obviously there is a need to channel our individuality into a productive force, and not allow it to run amok with no direction. But that is the challenge not of individuality, but of subjectivity; we must not allow our subjective selves to cloud our ethical judgment. However subjectivity should not be confused with individuality –– our Divine uniqueness that give us our indispensable mission in this universe. Here is my advice to you: If you want to be a true free spirit – and express your deepest individuality – return and learn to be a great teacher, to find what you were deprived of. Teach them the soul of mindfulness; teach them how to fly on its wings.

Apothecary Recipes

BEGIN TO LEARN AND BUILD YOUR APOTHECARY RECIPES.

Quick Start Apothecary Recipes for Beginners

Herbal Apothecary Cards

Sage Gargle

Sore throat • Hot flashes • Poor digestion

Herbal Apothecary Cards

STEEP 1 TABLESPOON DRIED SAGE LEAVES IN 1¼ CUPS OF JUST-BOILED WATER. LET STAND, COVERED, FOR 5 MINUTES, COVERED. STRAIN OFF THE LEAVES. ADD A PINCH OF SALT AND STIR TO DISSOLVE. USE AS A GARGLE FOR SORE THROAT.

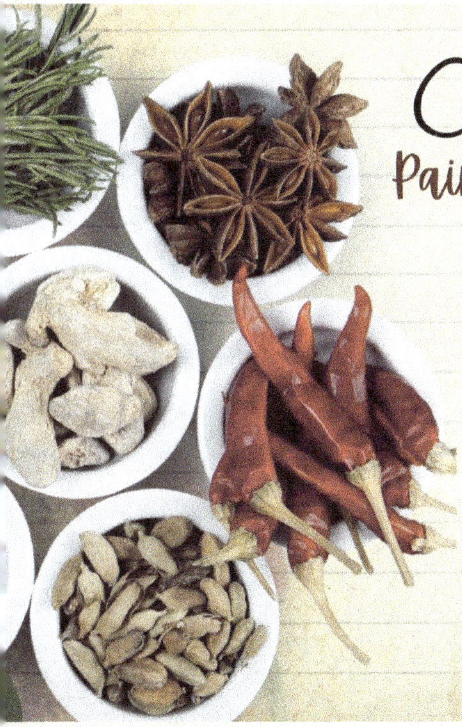

Cayenne Pepper
Pain • Poor circulation • External bleeding
Herbal Apothecary Cards

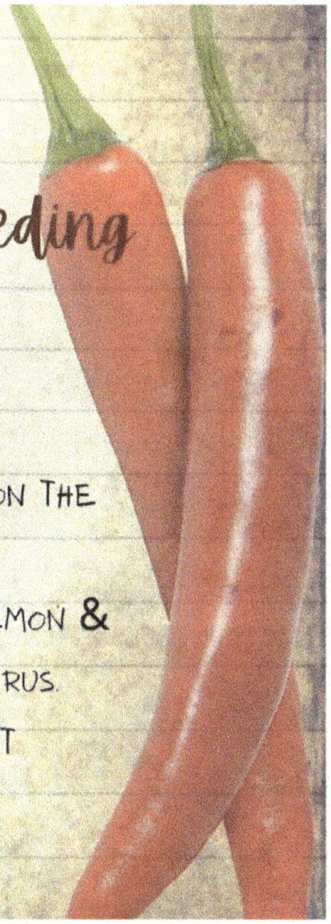

Cayenne pepper is a type of Capsicum annuum.
Three ways to use cayenne
1) For a small bleeding cut, sprinkle cayenne pepper on the cut to stop blood flow.
2) For a cold, add a pinch of cayenne to your ginger, lemon & honey tea. To help warm things up and kick that cold virus.
3) Some recommend 1 tablespoon of this to stop a heart attack

The Apothecary Farmacy

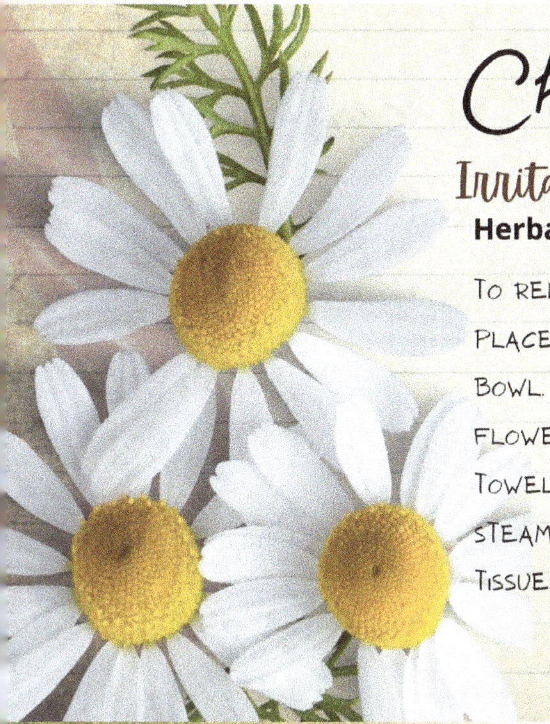

Chamomile
Irritability • Sleep issues • Cold and flu symptoms
Herbal Apothecary Cards

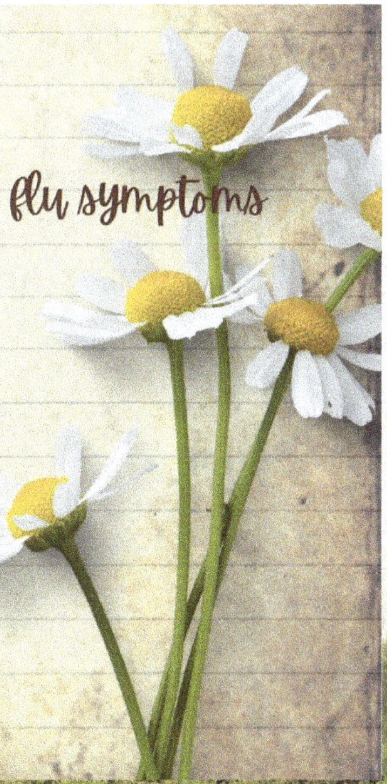

To relieve sinus congestion and inflammation, place a handful of chamomile in a mediumsized bowl. Pour just-boiled water over the flowers. Place your head over the bowl with a towel draped around your head to capture the steam. Do this for 10 minutes as needed. Keep tissues nearby to blow your nose as needed.

The Apothecary Farmacy

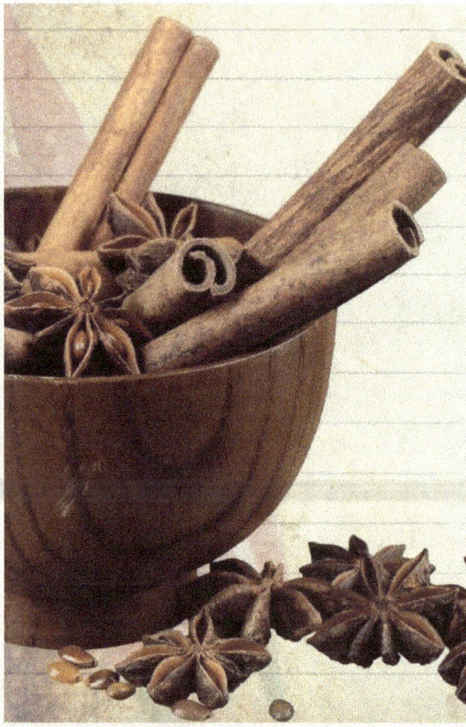

Cinnamon
Toothache • Diarrhea • Insulin resistance

Herbal Apothecary Cards

CINNAMON TOOTH POWDER

THIS IS A DELICIOUS WAY TO BRUSH YOUR TEETH AND KEEP YOUR GUMS HEALTHY. PLACE ½ TEASPOON OF CINNAMON POWDER ON A WET TOOTHBRUSH. BRUSH AS YOU NORMALLY WOULD.

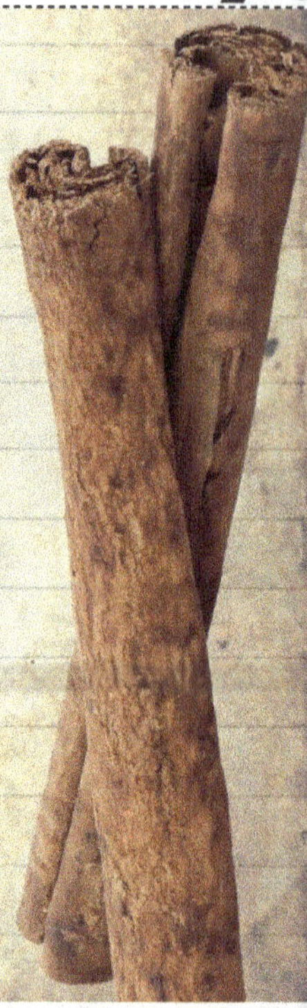

THE APOTHECARY FARMACY

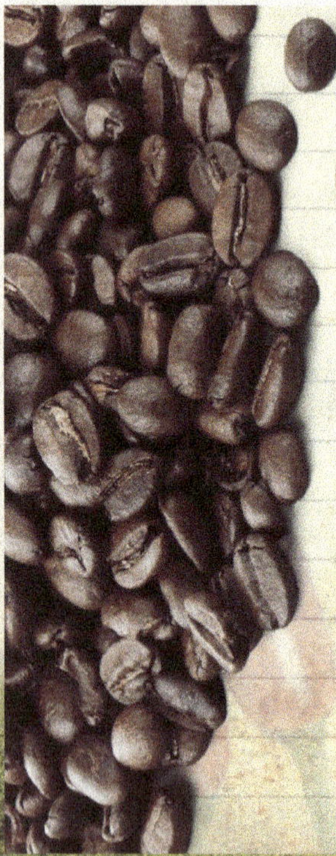

Spiced Cold Brew
Fatigue • Constipation • Contains antioxidants

Herbal Apothecary Cards

PLACE 1 CUP COARSELY GROUND COFFEE BEANS, ½ TEASPOON CINNAMON POWDER AND ¼ TEASPOON CARDAMOM POWDER INTO A 1-QUART JAR. FILL THE JAR WITH WATER AND STIR WELL. COVER AND STORE IN THE FRIDGE FOR 12 HOURS. STRAIN. TO DRINK, MIX ¼ CUP OF THE COFFEE BREW WITH ½ CUP WATER OR CREAM. ADD SWEETENER IF DESIRED. SERVE ON ICE. NOT A COFFEE DRINKER?

NOTE: COFFEE IS A USEFUL HERB IN MODERATION. ALSO SEE COFFEE ENEMA.

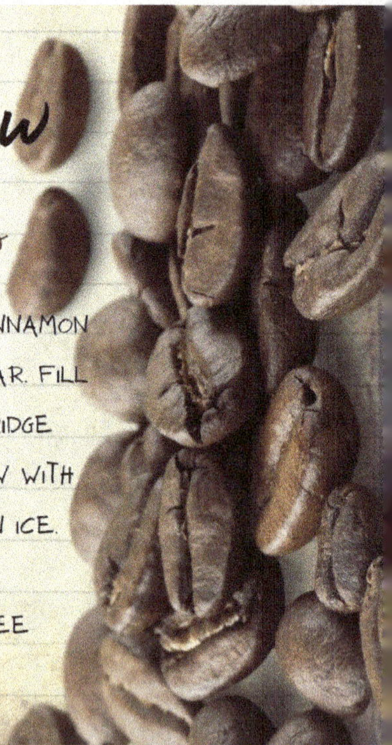

THE APOTHECARY FARMACY

Coffee Enema

Relieve Constipation • Boost Immunity • Increase Energy

Herbal Apothecary Cards

Use one quart of filtered water with one tablespoon to one cup of brewed, organic, air-roasted enema coffee for this colon-cleansing solution. Hold the coffee enema solution for 15 minutes after you have taken all of the coffee solution into your colon. Once the time has passed, empty your colon.

*** Gerson Therapy uses it to help cure diseases including cancer.

THE APOTHECARY FARMACY

Elderberry Syrup

Prevent or stop colds and flu • Inflammation

Herbal Apothecary Cards

Simmer 1 cup dried elderberries and 3 cups water in a small saucepan for 20 minutes. Strain off the berries through a cheesecloth, squeezing really well. Add 1 cup honey and stir well to dissolve. Store in the fridge. Adults take by the tablespoon. Kids (over 2) by the teaspoon. Use for regular immune health, as well as cold and flu symptoms.

THE APOTHECARY FARMACY

Fever Tea

Prevent or stop colds and flu • Fevers • Protect the skin

Herbal Apothecary Cards

Steep ½ cup dried elderflowers and 2 tablespoons dried peppermint in 2½ cups of just-boiled water. Let stand, covered, for 30 minutes. Strain. Add honey to taste. Drink warm or cold throughout the day.

THE APOTHECARY FARMACY

Dandelion Root Tea

Liver health • Acne • Poor digestion

Herbal Apothecary Cards

Simmer 1 tablespoon roasted dandelion roots in 1½ cups water for 20 minutes. Strain. Add honey and/or cream as desired. Purchasing roasted roots is a great introduction to using this safe and nourishing herb. Do not gather wild—

THE APOTHECARY FARMACY

Cracked Pepper

Absorption • Mucus congestion • Poor circulation

Herbal Apothecary Cards

Add to your turmeric or ghee; sprinkle freshly ground pepper on all meals to increase bioavailability in your meal. That's right – you can absorb more nutrients from your meal with this tasty spice.

THE APOTHECARY FARMACY

Peppermint

Upset stomach • Headache • Skin itching and inflammation

Herbal Apothecary Cards

Add ¼ cup peppermint leaves to 1 cup of just-boiled water. Let stand, covered, for 10 minutes. Strain off the leaves and reserve the liquid. Soak a washcloth in the liquid and squeeze to remove excess liquid. Apply to forehead to relieve a headache or to skin to relieve itching and inflammation.

THE APOTHECARY FARMACY

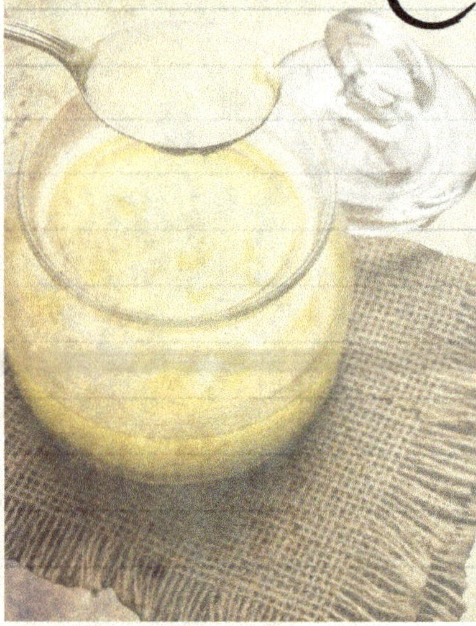

Curry Powder Ghee

Inflammation • Poor digestion • Pain

Herbal Apothecary Cards

Mix together 2 tablespoons cumin powder, 2 tablespoons coriander powder, 1 tablespoon turmeric powder, 1½ teaspoons cinnamon powder, ¾ teaspoon clove powder, ¾ teaspoon cardamom powder and heat ghee and stir inside your ghee

THE APOTHECARY FARMACY

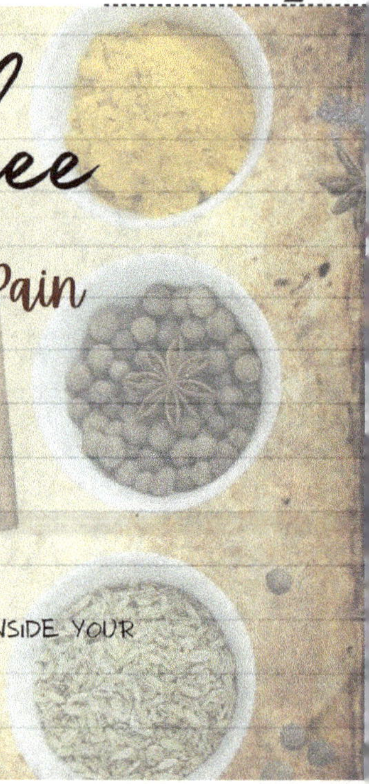

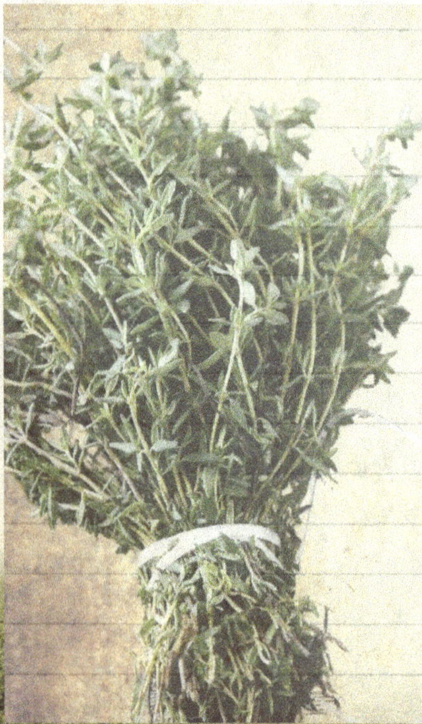

Thyme Tea

Coughs • Congestion • Infections

Herbal Apothecary Cards

Steep 1 tablespoon dried thyme in 1¼ cups of just-boiled water. Let stand, covered, for 5 minutes. Strain off the leaves. Add honey to taste. Use to address coughs, congestion and sore throats.

THE APOTHECARY FARMACY

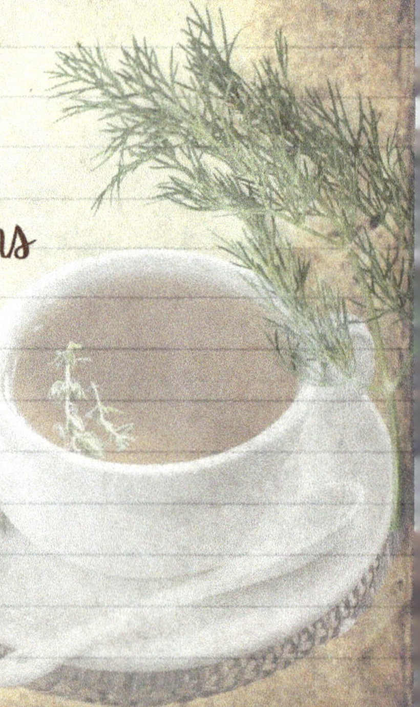

Ginger, Lemon & Honey Tea

Nausea • Cold and flu symptoms • Inflammation

Herbal Apothecary Cards

CUT OFF THE ENDS. STEAM FOR 15 MINUTES. DRY IN THE SUN FOR 4 HOURS. PUT IN A JAR, COVER WITH ORGANIC RAW HONEY AND PUT IN THE REFRIGERATOR. EAT IN YOUR LETTUCE WRAPS OR JUST EAT. READY IN 24 HOURS. EAT 3-7 A DAY FOR 7 DAYS. FOR BETTER RESULTS LET FERMENT 5-7 DAYS.

THE APOTHECARY FARMACY

Immune System

Herbal Apothecary Cards

- CAYENNE
- CHAI
- CHAMOMILE
- CINNAMON
- ECHINACEA
- ELDERBERRY
- ELDERFLOWER
- PEPPERMINT
- SAGE
- GINGER

Ashwagandha, reishi (both of which stimulate your infection fighting lymphocytes, or white blood cells,) and holy basil (stimulates the immune system and also fights viruses) are all good choices for immune support, Try mixing reishi, Ashwagandha, and a few items from the list as a powder and mix it into anything you're eating or drinking to boost your immune system.

THE APOTHECARY FARMACY

Temperature
Herbal Apothecary Cards

- CAYENNE
- CHAI
- CINNAMON
- ELDERFLOWER
- GARLIC
- GINGER
- PEPPER
- SAGE
- THYME

The herb **feverfew** derives its name from its reported ability to reduce fevers. **Chamomile, yarrow, elderflower** and **lemon balm** herbs also induce perspiration, which may help bring down body temperature. Provided is a list of herbs to help with a fever.

THE APOTHECARY FARMACY

Digestion
Herbal Apothecary Cards

- CAYENNE
- CHAMOMILE
- CINNAMON
- DANDELION
- GARLIC
- GINGER
- PEPPERMINT
- SAGE
- THYME
- TURMERIC

In TCM, these issues are traditionally treated with digestive tonic herbs such as **Chinese Yam** (also known as Mountain Yam), **Wild Cardamom, Atractylodes** and **Codonopsis**, which work together to harmonise Stomach and Spleen functions and improve the breakdown of food, uptake and transformation of nutrients and Qi, and elimination of wastes.

THE APOTHECARY FARMACY

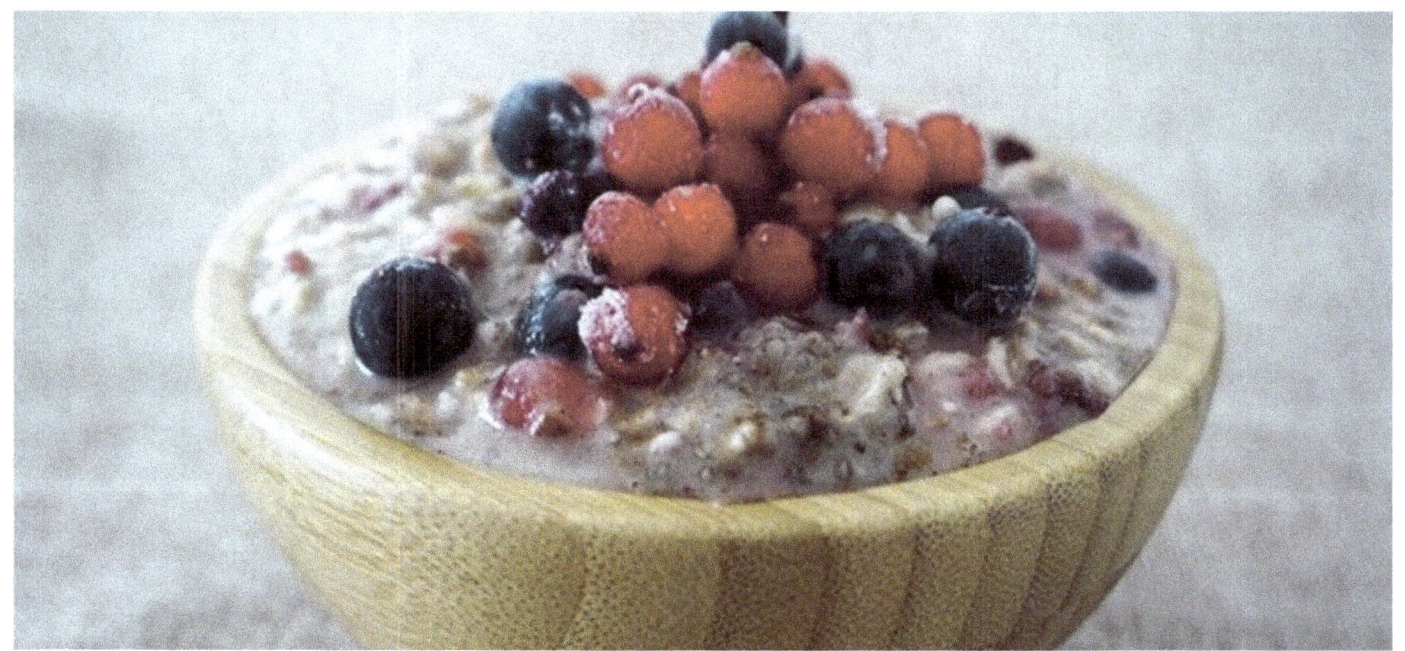

Berry Oats

Preparation Time: 10 minutes / Cooking Time: 8 minutes
Serves: 3

Ingredients

½ cup rolled oats
2 cup coconut milk
1 pinch sea salt
1 pinch cinnamon powder
3 tbsp maple syrup
½ cup blueberries
4 tbsp wild berries
1 tbsp coconut butter

Nutrition Facts

Servings:	3
Amount per serving	
Calories	533
Total Fat	42.2g
Saturated Fat	36.7g
Cholesterol	0mg
Sodium	107mg
Total Carbohydrate	39.7g
Dietary Fiber	6.9g
Total Sugars	22.5g
Protein	6.2g

Instructions

♦ In a saucepan, add the coconut butter, rolled oats and coconut milk.

♦ Stir well and cook until it comes to boil.

♦ Add the salt, cinnamon, and maple syrup.

♦ Simmer until it thickens.

♦ Take off the heat and let it cool down.

♦ Fold in the berries and mix well. Serve in room temperature or cold.

Total Fat 42.2g 54%
Saturated Fat 36.7g 183%
Cholesterol 0mg 0%
Sodium 107mg 5%
Total Carbohydrate 39.7g 14%
Dietary Fiber 6.9g 25%

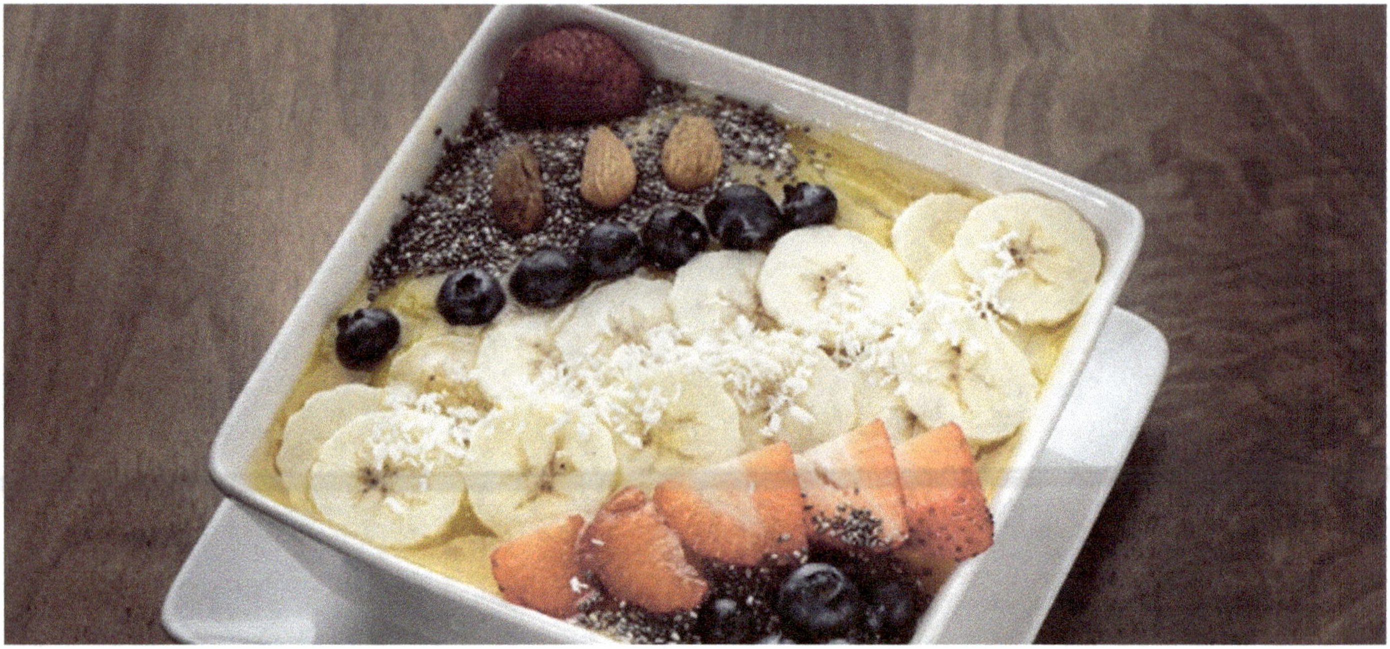

Turmeric Banana Berry Smoothie Bowl

Preparation Time: 5 minutes
Serves: 2

Ingredients

1 cup almond milk
4 ice cubes
¼ tsp turmeric
2 ripe banana, sliced
½ cup strawberries, diced
1 pinch sea salt
2 tbsp blueberries
3 almonds
1 tbsp chia seeds

Nutrition Facts

Servings:	2
Amount per serving	
Calories	611
Total Fat	41.9g
Saturated Fat	26.9g
Cholesterol	0mg
Sodium	144mg
Total Carbohydrate	56.3g
Dietary Fiber	22.3g
Total Sugars	21.1g
Protein	11.5g

Instructions

♦ Reserve some of the banana slices and strawberries to use later.

♦ In a blender, pour the almond milk.

♦ Add the ice cubes, sea salt, banana slices, strawberries, turmeric, and blend for 2 minutes.

♦ Add to two bowls.

♦ Top with chia seeds, blueberries, almonds, banana slices, and strawberries. Serve.

Total Fat 41.9g
54%

Saturated Fat 26.9g
135%

Cholesterol 0mg
0%

Sodium 144mg

Total Carbohydrate 56.3g

Dietary Fiber 22.3g

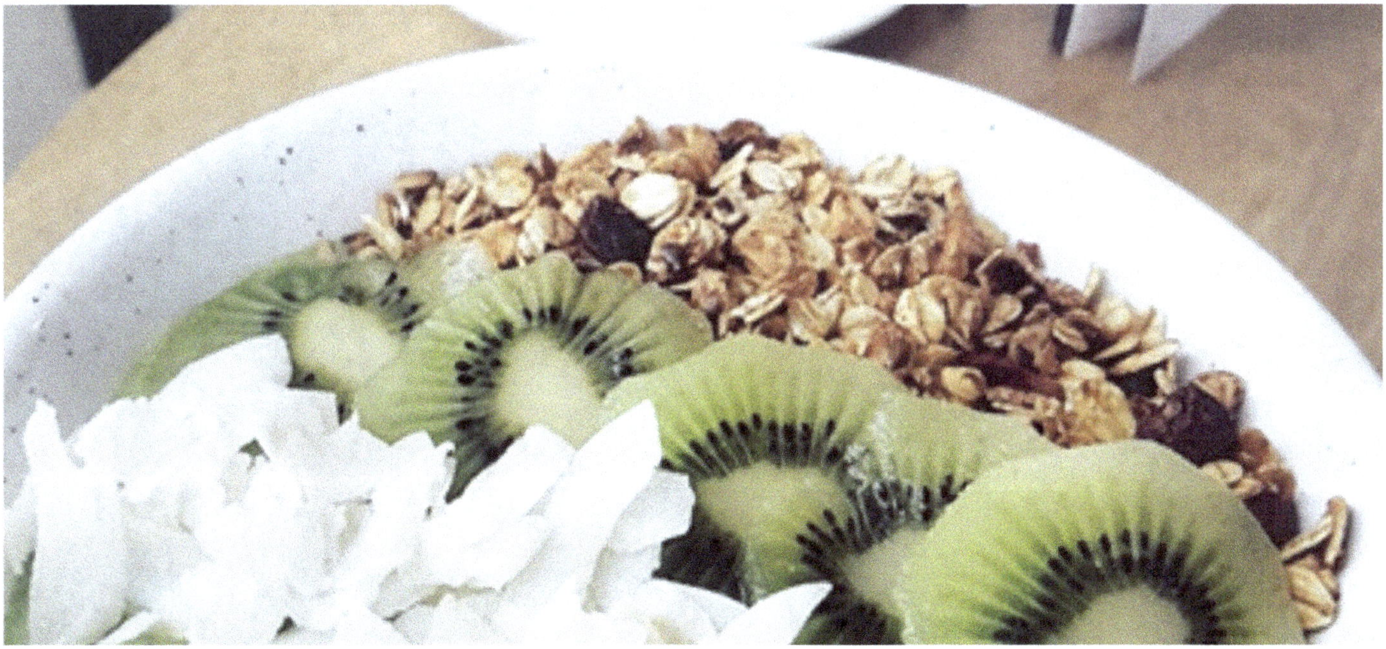

Avocado Coconut Kiwi Smoothie Bowl

Preparation Time: 5 minutes
Serves: 2

Ingredients

1 cup coconut milk
½ cup kiwi, sliced
1 cup ripe avocado cubes
1 pinch sea salt
2 tbsp coconut flakes
2 tbsp granola, toasted
1 tbsp currants
4 ice cubes
1 tbsp peppermint

Nutrition Facts

Servings:	2
Amount per serving	
Calories	494
Total Fat	48.8g
Saturated Fat	30.6g
Cholesterol	0mg
Sodium	147mg
Total Carbohydrate	29.2g
Dietary Fiber	11.2g
Total Sugars	12g
Protein	7.3g

Instructions

- Reserve some kiwi slices to add as topping later.
- In a blender, combine the coconut milk.
- Add the avocado cubes, kiwi, peppermint, salt, ice cubes and blend for 90 seconds.
- Pour into two bowls.
- Top with granola, kiwi slices, coconut flakes and currants. Serve.

Total Fat 48.8g 63%
Saturated Fat 30.6g 153%
Cholesterol 0mg
0%

Sodium 147mg 6%
Total Carbohydrate 29.2g 11%
Dietary Fiber 11.2g 40%

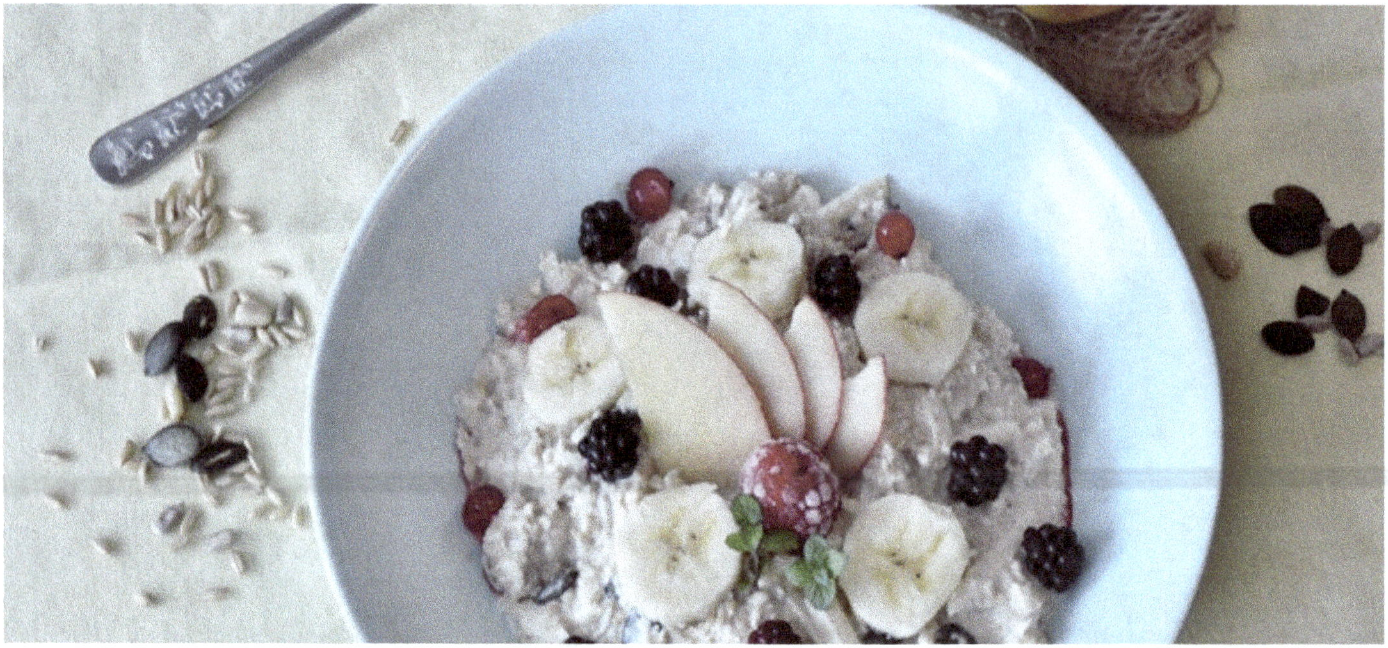

Overnight Oats with Fruits and Nuts

Preparation Time: 8 hours
Serves: 3

Ingredients

½ cup rolled oats
2 cup almond milk
½ half banana, mashed
½ banana slices
1 pinch sea salt
2 tbsp maple syrup
2 tbsp wild berries
2 tbsp blackberries
½ apple, sliced lengthwise

Nutrition Facts

Servings:	3
Amount per serving	
Calories	508
Total Fat	39.7g
Saturated Fat	34.1g
Cholesterol	0mg
Sodium	115mg
Total Carbohydrate	39.2g
Dietary Fiber	6.9g
Total Sugars	21.1g
Protein	6.6g

Instructions

- In a bowl, add the rolled oats with the almond milk.
- Add the mashed banana and whisk well.
- Add the maple syrup, sea salt, and mix well.
- Cover with a lid and fridge it for 8 hours.
- Serve with apples, bananas, wild berries and blackberries.

Total Fat 39.7g 51%

Saturated Fat 34.1g 171%

Cholesterol 0mg
0%

Sodium 115mg 5%

Total Carbohydrate 39.2g 14%

Dietary Fiber 6.9g 25%

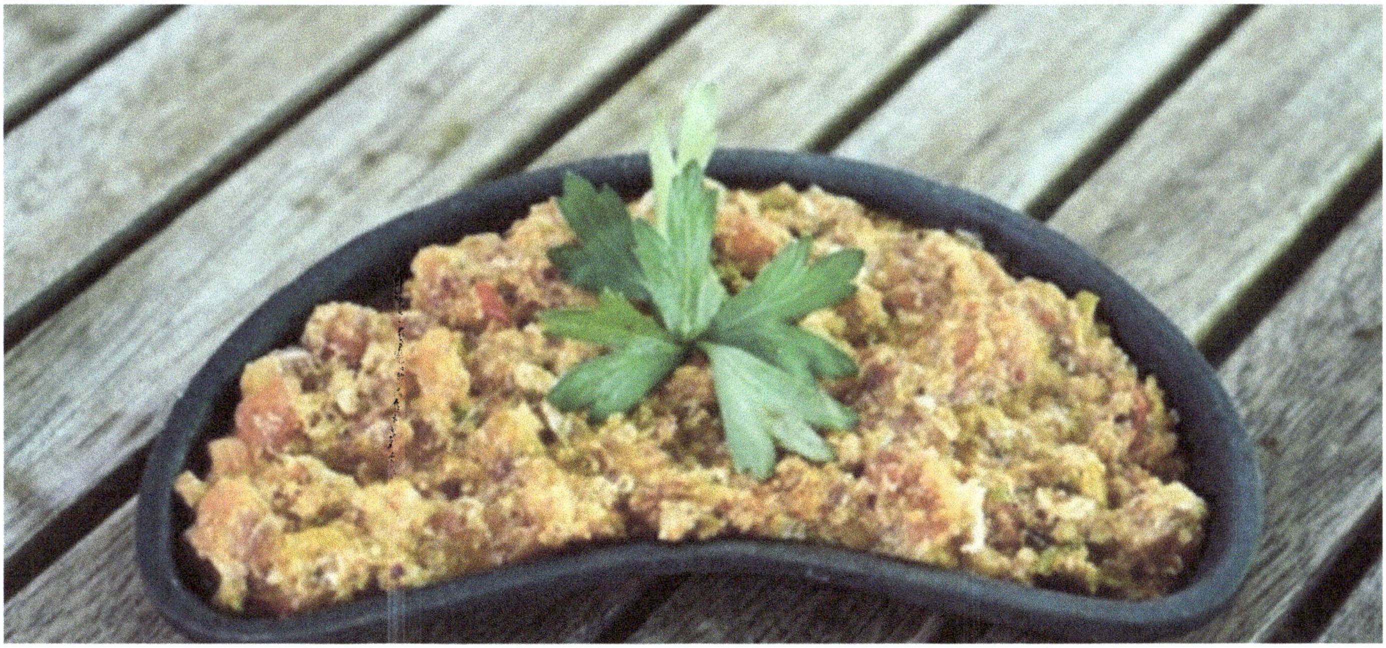

Tofu Tomato Garlic Scramble

Preparation Time: 5 minutes / Cooking Time: 8 minutes
Serves: 2

Ingredients

- 1 cup soft tofu, crumbled
- 1 onion, chopped
- 2 tomatoes, chopped
- 4 garlic cloves, minced
- ½ tsp cumin
- Salt and pepper to taste
- ¼ tsp ginger powder
- 1 tsp tahini
- 1 tsp parsley, chopped
- 2 tsp oil
- ½ tsp paprika

Nutrition Facts

Servings:	2
Amount per serving	
Calories	188
Total Fat	11g
Saturated Fat	1.5g
Cholesterol	0mg
Sodium	24mg
Total Carbohydrate	15.4g
Dietary Fiber	3.6g
Total Sugars	6.6g
Protein	10.8g

Instructions

- In a skillet, add the oil over medium heat.
- Add the garlic and cook for 1 minute.
- Add the onion, and toss until it becomes golden.
- Add the tomatoes and stir for 2 minutes.
- Add the crumbled tofu and stir for 1 minute.
- Add the cumin, salt, pepper, ginger powder, tahini, and paprika.
- Stir for 3 minutes and add the parsley. Take off the heat.
- Serve hot.

Total Fat 11g
14%

Saturated Fat 1.5g
8%

Cholesterol 0mg
0%

Sodium 24mg
1%

Total Carbohydrate 15.4g
6%

Dietary Fiber 3.6g
13%

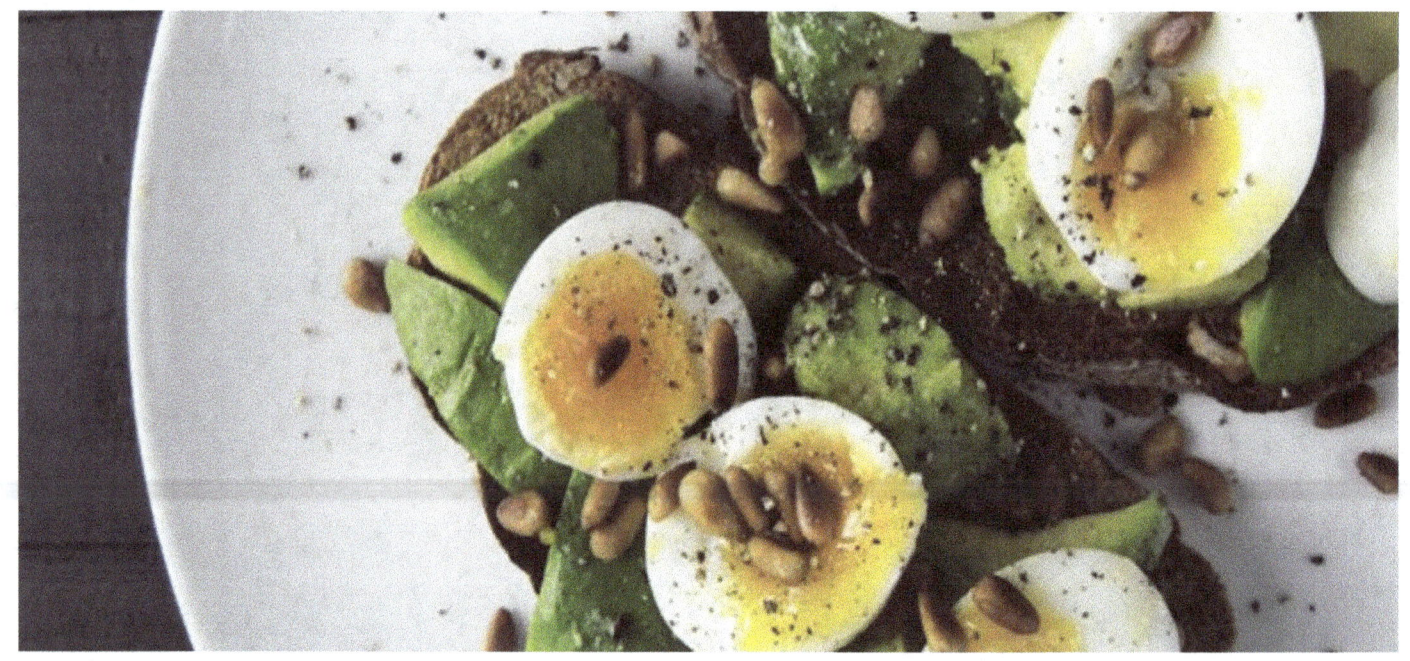

Avocado Egg Toast

Preparation Time: 5 minutes / Cooking Time: 8 minutes
Serves: 2

Ingredients

2 brown bread slices
2 eggs
3 tbsp pine nuts, toasted
1 semi ripe avocado, diced
½ tsp cumin
Salt and pepper to taste
2 tsp olive oil

Nutrition Facts

Servings:	2
Amount per serving	
Calories	485
Total Fat	38.3g
Saturated Fat	6.9g
Cholesterol	164mg
Sodium	353mg
Total Carbohydrate	30.4g
Dietary Fiber	9.4g
Total Sugars	2.4g
Protein	11.7g

Instructions

- Boil the eggs in salted water for 5 minutes.
- Drain and add to a cold bath.
- Remove the shells and cut into slices.
- Toast the bread slices and add the avocado pieces.
- Add the egg slices, pine nuts, salt, pepper, cumin and olive oil on top. Serve.

Total Fat 38.3g 49%

Saturated Fat 6.9g 35%

Cholesterol 164mg 55%

Sodium 353mg 15%

Total Carbohydrate 30.4g 11%

Dietary Fiber 9.4g 34%

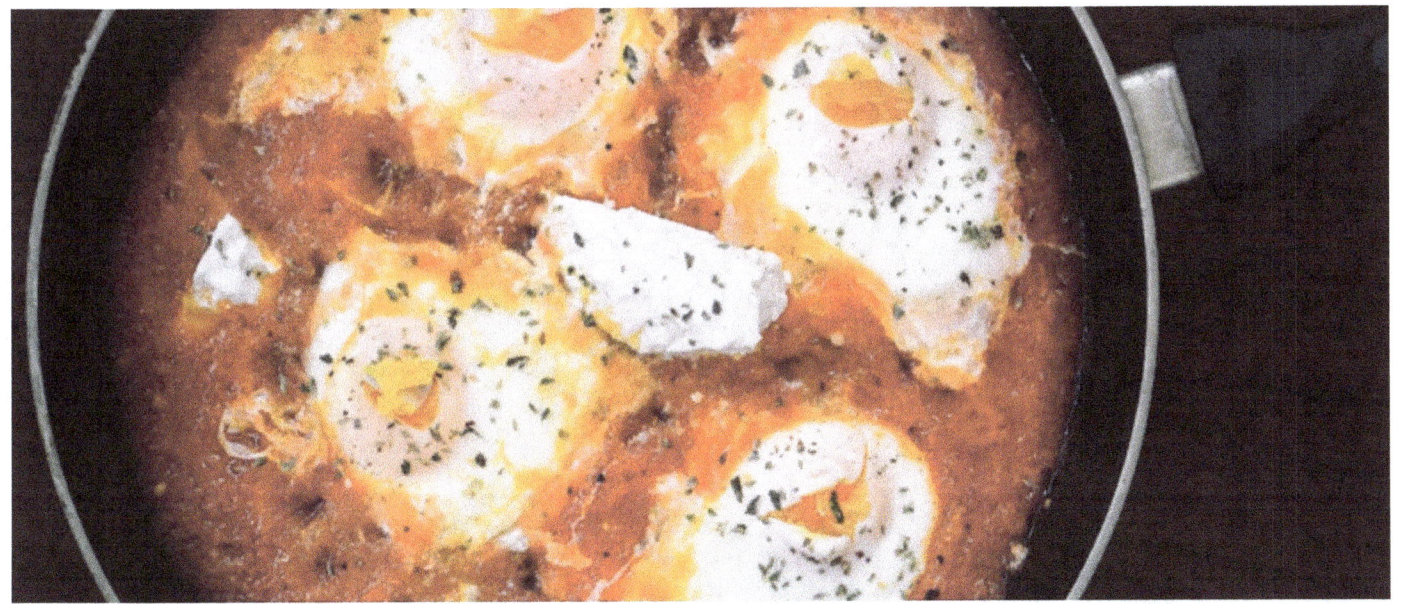

Delicious Shaksuka

Preparation Time: 10 minutes / Cooking Time: 20 minutes
Serves: 4

Ingredients

4 eggs
2 tablespoons olive oil
1 red bell pepper, chopped
1 onion, chopped
¼ teaspoon sea salt
2 tablespoons tomato paste
3 cloves garlic, minced
1 teaspoon cumin
¼ teaspoon chili flakes
½ teaspoon smoked paprika
1 cup crushed tomatoes
2 tablespoon cilantro, chopped
Black pepper to taste
½ cup crumbled feta

Nutrition Facts

Servings:	4
Amount per serving	
Calories	231
Total Fat	15.7g
Saturated Fat	5.2g
Cholesterol	180mg
Sodium	519mg
Total Carbohydrate	13.6g
Dietary Fiber	3.6g
Total Sugars	8.3g
Protein	10.9g

Instructions

- In a large skillet, add the olive oil over medium heat.
- Add the garlic and onion and fry for 1 minute.
- Add the crushed tomatoes and toss for 2 minutes.
- Add the bell pepper and toss for 2 minutes.
- Add the salt, cumin, paprika, pepper, chili flakes, tomato paste and cook for 3 minutes.
- Break the egg in the middle and cover with lid.
- Cook for 5 minutes. Sprinkle some more salt and pepper on top.
- Add the feta, cilantro on top. Serve hot.

Total Fat 15.7g 20%

Saturated Fat 5.2g 26%

Cholesterol 180mg 60%

Sodium 519mg 23%

Total Carbohydrate 13.6g 5%

Dietary Fiber 3.6g 13%

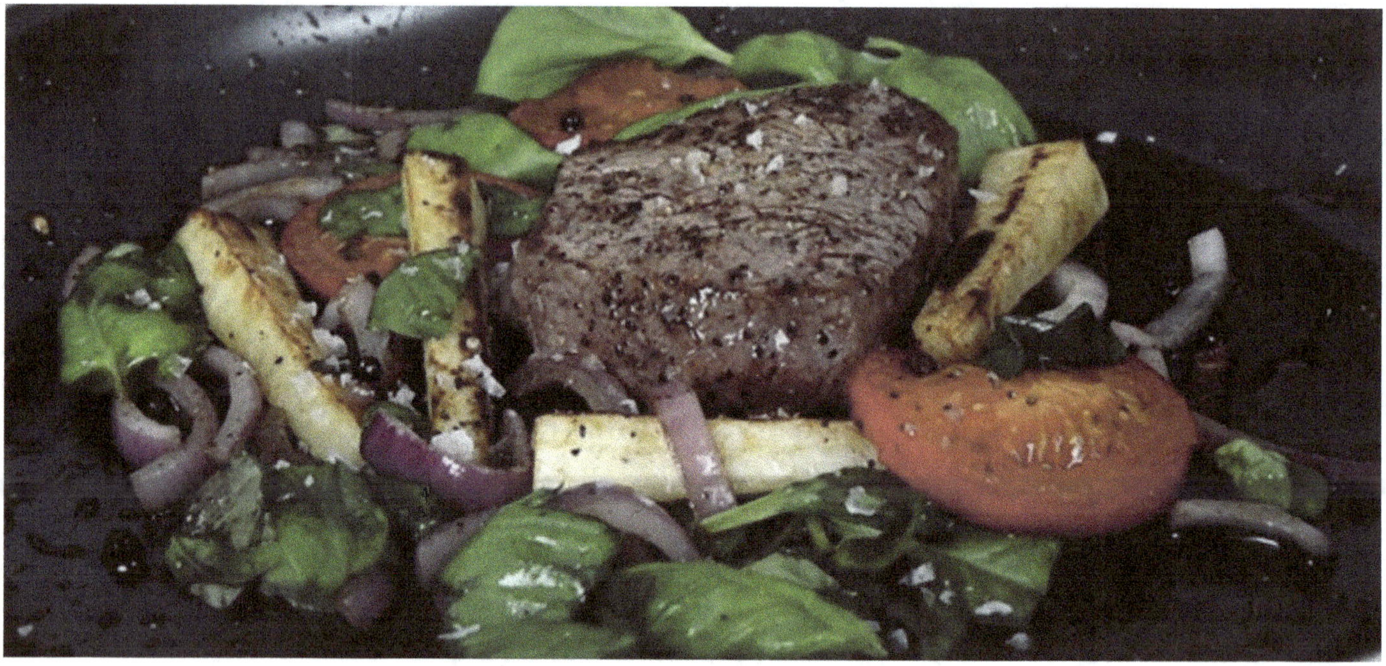

Beef Steak with Vegetables

Preparation Time: 10 minutes / Cooking Time: 12 minutes
Serves: 1

Ingredients

1 beef steak
½ plantains cut into 2 inch lengthwise strips
1 tomato, cut into wedges
1 red onion, sliced
½ cup basil leaves
Salt and pepper to taste
1 tbsp olive oil
½ tsp garlic powder
½ tsp ginger powder
1 tsp soy sauce

Nutrition Facts

Servings:	1
Amount per serving	
Calories	456
Total Fat	20g
Saturated Fat	4.2g
Cholesterol	76mg
Sodium	367mg
Total Carbohydrate	43.7g
Dietary Fiber	5.7g
Total Sugars	20.2g
Protein	29.8g

Instructions

♦ Marinate the beef steak with garlic, ginger, salt, pepper, and soy sauce for 10 minutes.

♦ In a pan, add the steak and cook for 4 minutes.

♦ Add the vegetables around the steam.

♦ Flip the steak and stir the vegetables. Sprinkle some salt, pepper on top.

♦ Cook for another 5 minutes. Take off the heat. Let it rest for 10 minutes.

♦ Serve.

Total Fat 20g
26%

Saturated Fat 4.2g
21%

Cholesterol 76mg
25%

Sodium 367mg
16%

Total Carbohydrate 43.7g
16%

Dietary Fiber 5.7g
20%

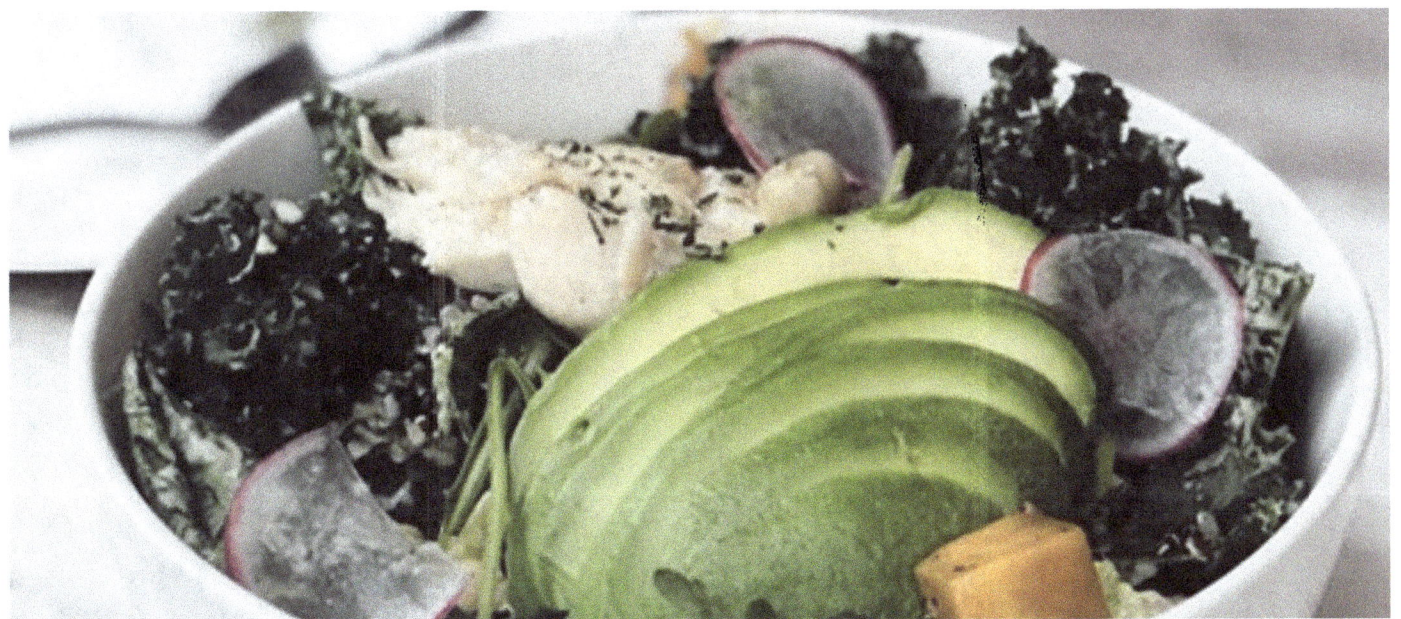

Kale Squash Avocado Radish Salad

Preparation Time: 5 minutes / Cooking Time: 10 minutes
Serves: 2

Ingredients

½ cup squash cubes
1 cup kale, roughly chopped
4 tbsp baby arugula
1 radish, sliced thinly
1 tsp sesame oil
½ avocado, sliced thickly
Salt and pepper to taste
½ tsp dill, minced
¼ tsp ginger, minced
1 tbsp olive oil
3 garlic cloves, sliced
2 tbsp apple cider vinegar
1 tsp black cumin seeds
2 tbsp garlic mayo

Nutrition Facts

Servings:	2
Amount per serving	
Calories	280
Total Fat	24.7g
Saturated Fat	4.2g
Cholesterol	5mg
Sodium	59mg
Total Carbohydrate	15g
Dietary Fiber	4.9g
Total Sugars	1.3g
Protein	2.9g

Instructions

- In a skillet, add half of the olive oil.
- Add the squash cubes and some salt, and pepper.
- Stir for about 5 minutes. Take off the heat. Let it cool down.
- In a large bowl, combine the arugula with kale, squash, and radish slices.
- Add the avocado slices on top.
- In a small container, mix together the lime juice, salt, sesame oil, pepper, apple cider vinegar, ginger, and garlic.
- Add the dressing onto the salad. Add the garlic mayo and dill on top. Serve fresh.

Total Fat 24.7g
32%

Saturated Fat 4.2g
21%

Cholesterol 5mg
2%

Sodium 59mg
3%

Total Carbohydrate 15g
5%

Dietary Fiber 4.9g
18%

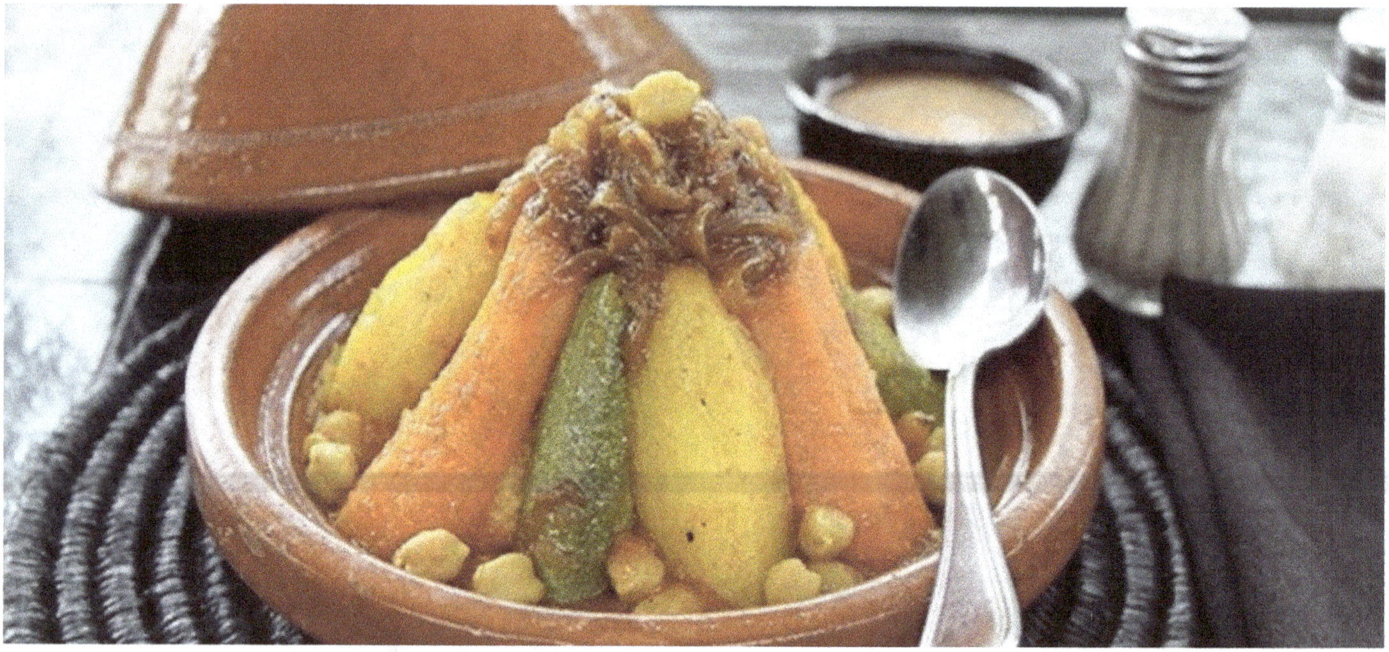

Chickpea Vegetable Curry

Preparation Time: 5 minutes / Cooking Time: 20 minutes
Serves: 4

Ingredients

1 cup chickpeas, boiled
1 cup zucchini, cut roughly lengthwise
1 cup carrots cut roughly lengthwise
2 inch ginger, minced
½ cup onion, chopped
Salt and pepper to taste
1 tsp paprika
1 tbsp olive oil
4 garlic cloves, sliced
1 tsp cumin
½ tsp dried oregano
1 cup vegetable stock
1 tsp coriander powder

Nutrition Facts

Servings:	4
Amount per serving	
Calories	243
Total Fat	6.9g
Saturated Fat	0.9g
Cholesterol	0mg
Sodium	46mg
Total Carbohydrate	36.9g
Dietary Fiber	10.6g
Total Sugars	7.8g
Protein	10.9g

Instructions

- In a saucepan, add the olive oil. Add the onion and cook for 2 minutes.
- Stir in the ginger and garlic and cook for a minute.
- Add the spices, and pour in the vegetable stock.
- Cook on high heat until it comes to boil.
- Stir in the vegetables and the chickpeas.
- Add the lid and simmer for 15 minutes. Serve hot.

Total Fat 6.9g
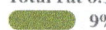 9%

Saturated Fat 0.9g
 4%

Cholesterol 0mg
0%

Sodium 46mg
 2%

Total Carbohydrate 36.9g
13%

Dietary Fiber 10.6g
38%

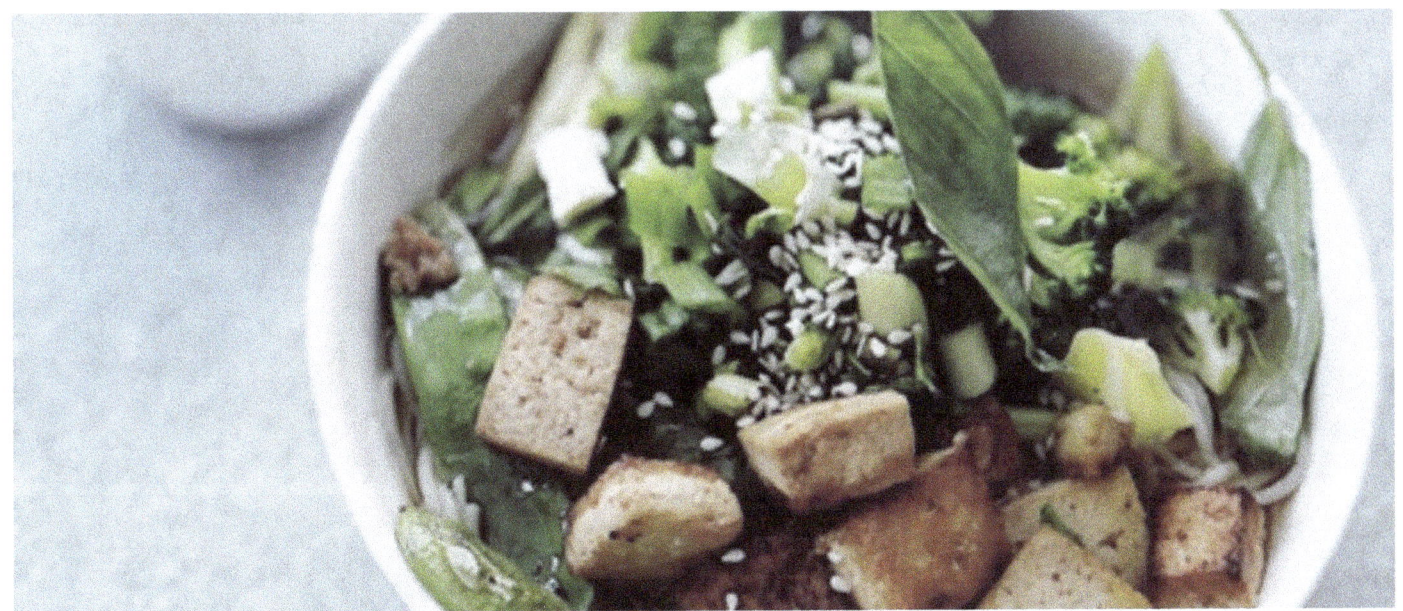

Tofu Snap Peas Broccoli Noodle Salad

Preparation Time: 5 minutes / Cooking Time: 10 minutes
Serves: 4

Ingredients

1 cup tofu cubes
1 cup rice noodles
½ cup collard leaves, chopped
½ cup snap peas
1 tbsp sesame seeds
½ cup broccoli, chopped roughly
2 tbsp scallions, chopped
Salt and pepper to taste
1/3 tsp rosemary, minced
1 tbsp olive oil
1 tsp garlic, minced
1 tbsp stevia
1 tsp ginger, minced
1 tbsp lime juice

Nutrition Facts

Servings:	4
Amount per serving	
Calories	140
Total Fat	6.1g
Saturated Fat	1g
Cholesterol	0mg
Sodium	15mg
Total Carbohydrate	16.9g
Dietary Fiber	2.8g
Total Sugars	1.4g
Protein	4.9g

Instructions

- In a saucepan, add the noodles with salted water.
- Cook for only 5 minutes. Drain and then let it cool down completely.
- In a skillet, add your oil over medium heat.
- Fry the tofu cubes for 5 minutes.
- Transfer to a kitchen tissue.
- In a bowl, combine the vegetables, rice noodles, tofu, and toss well.
- In a small bowl, mix together the lime juice, stevia, rosemary, salt, pepper, and sesame oil.
- Add on top of the salad. Add the sesame seeds on top. Serve.

Total Fat 6.1g
 8%

Saturated Fat 1g
5%

Cholesterol 0mg
0%

Sodium 15mg
 1%

Total Carbohydrate 16.9g
6%

Dietary Fiber 2.8g
10%

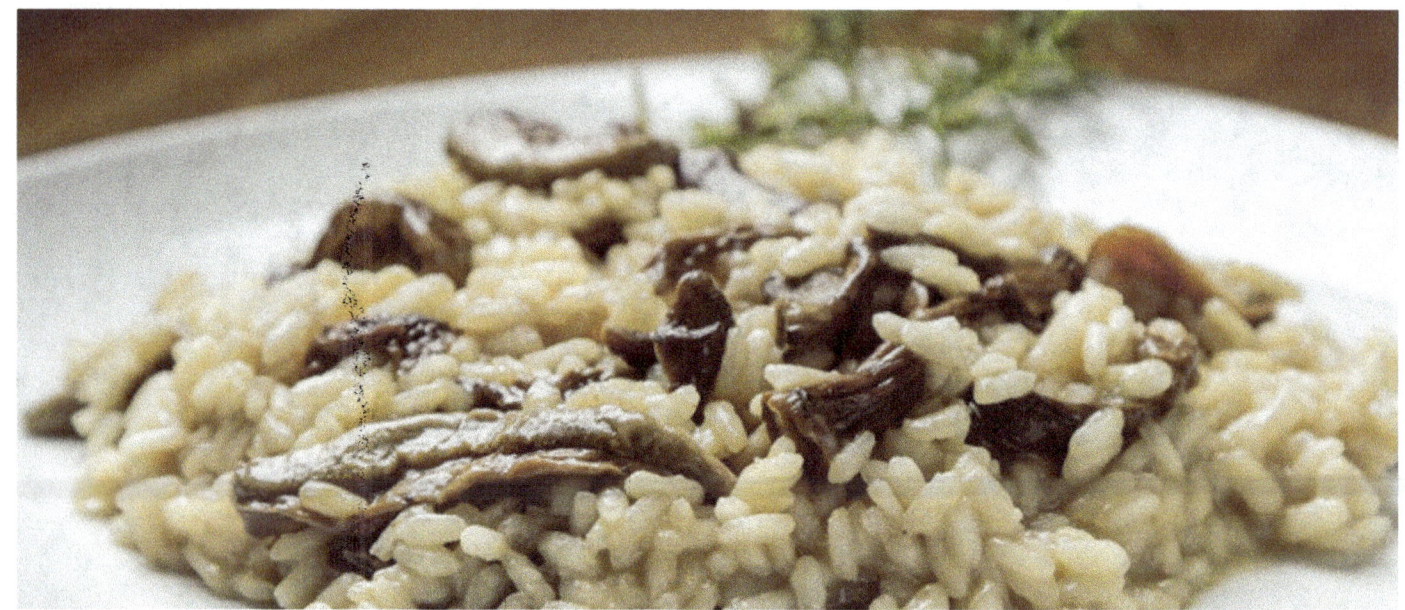

Mushroom Rosemary Garlic Risotto

Preparation Time: 5 minutes / Cooking Time: 25 minutes
Serves: 4

Ingredients

3 cup sticky rice
1 tbsp rosemary, minced
1 cup mixed mushrooms, sliced roughly
2 tsp garlic, minced
Salt to taste
1 tsp ginger, paste
White pepper to taste
6 cup mushroom stock
½ tsp dried oregano
1 tbsp almond butter

Nutrition Facts

Servings:	4
Amount per serving	
Calories	320
Total Fat	7.7g
Saturated Fat	1.8g
Cholesterol	1mg
Sodium	2435mg
Total Carbohydrate	57.7g
Dietary Fiber	5.6g
Total Sugars	1.4g
Protein	7.6g

Instructions

- Melt the almond butter in a saucepan.
- Add the garlic and cook until it becomes brown.
- Stir in the rice, ginger paste, and sauté for about 3 minutes.
- Stir in the mushroom, spices, and herbs.
- Toss for about 2 minutes and pour the stock.
- Stir and then add the lid.
- Cook on medium high heat for about 20 minutes.
- Sprinkle some more salt, pepper and the rosemary.
- Cook for 2 more and take off the heat. Serve warm.

Total Fat 7.7g
10%

Saturated Fat 1.8g
9%

Cholesterol 1mg
0%

Sodium 2435mg
106%

Total Carbohydrate 57.7g
21%

Dietary Fiber 5.6g
20%

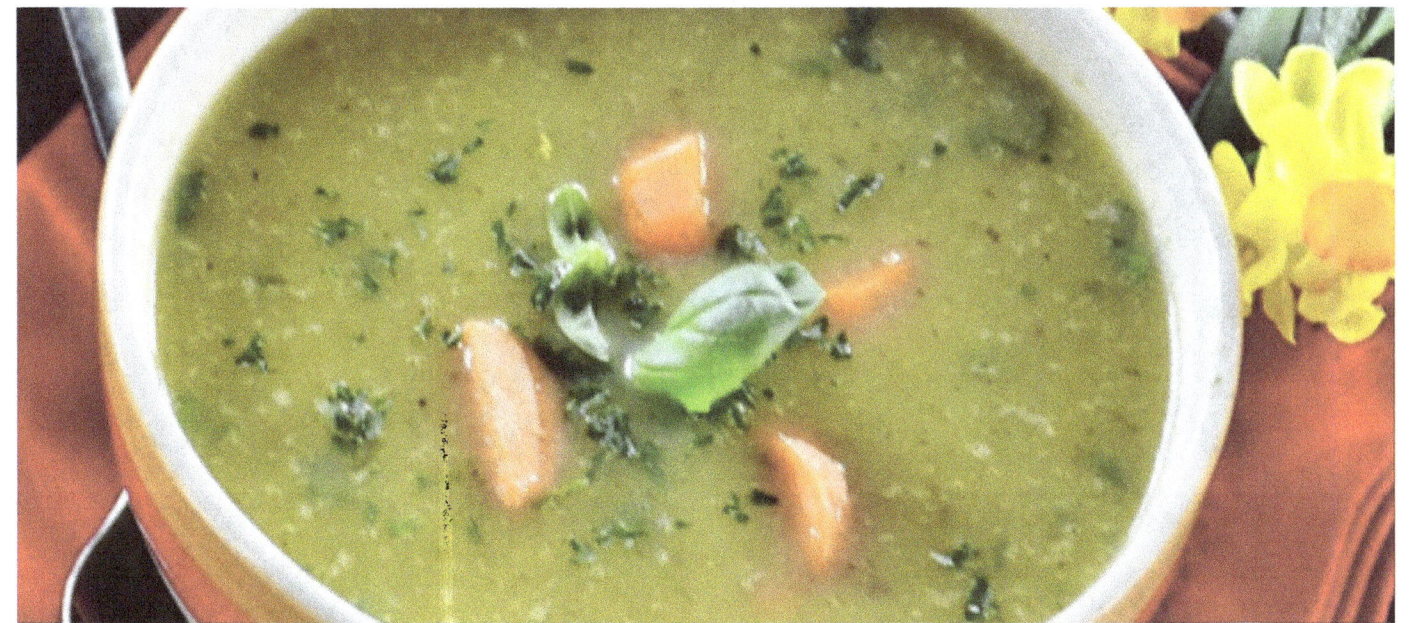

Lentil Soup

Preparation Time: 5 minutes / Cooking Time: 25 minutes
Serves: 2

Ingredients

1 cup red lentils
1 carrot, pureed
3 cup water
1 pinch turmeric
1 tsp garlic, minced
1 baby shallot, minced
1 tsp olive oil
Salt to taste
2 tbsp basil leaves, chopped
Carrot cubes to garnish, (optional)

Nutrition Facts

Servings:	2
Amount per serving	
Calories	378
Total Fat	3.4g
Saturated Fat	0.5g
Cholesterol	0mg
Sodium	116mg
Total Carbohydrate	62.1g
Dietary Fiber	30.1g
Total Sugars	3.5g
Protein	25.3g

Instructions

- In a saucepan, add the water and lentils.
- Cook on high heat for 10 minutes.
- Add the carrot puree, salt, turmeric, and simmer for 5 minutes.
- In another pan, add the olive oil over medium heat.
- Add the shallot and garlic and cook until they are golden.
- Add the onion mix into the lentil mix.
- Cook for 5 minutes. Use a hand blender and blend the mix until smooth.
- Add the basil on top and serve. You can use carrot cubes to garnish as well.
- Melt the almond butter in a saucepan.

Total Fat 3.4g
4%

Saturated Fat 0.5g
2%

Cholesterol 0mg
0%

Sodium 116mg
5%

Total Carbohydrate 62.1g
23%

Dietary Fiber 30.1g
108%

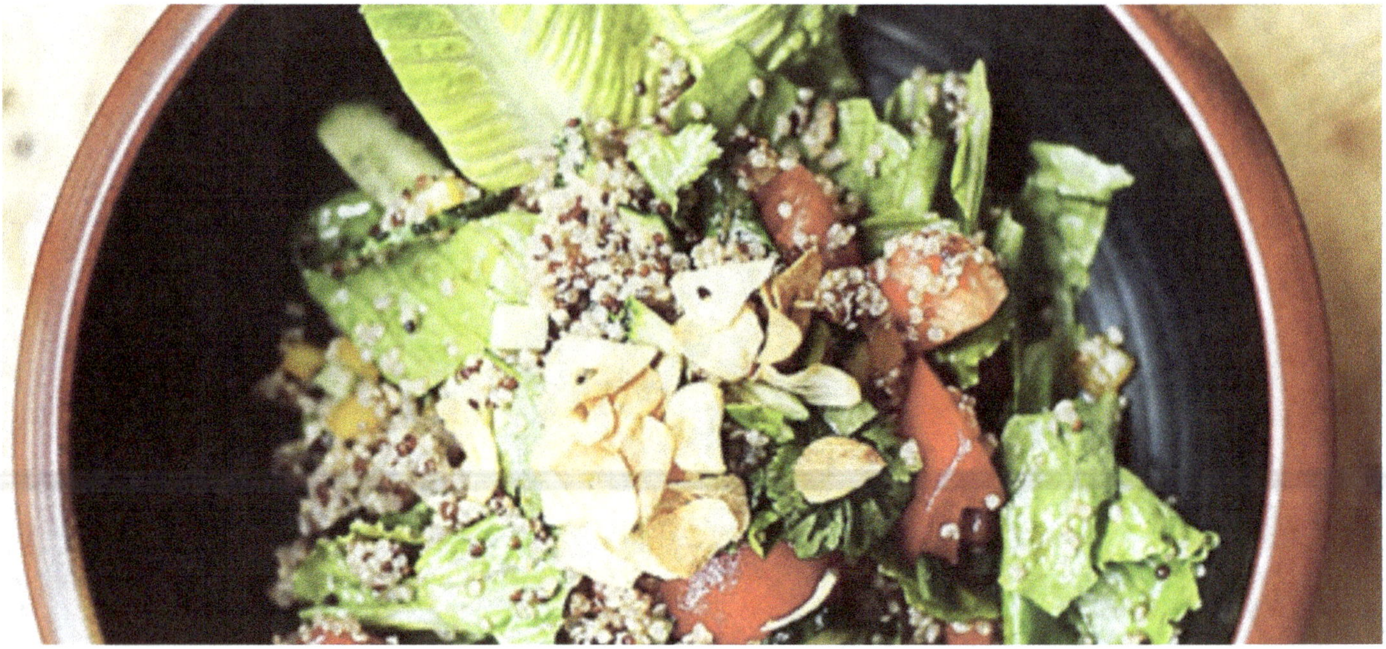

Couscous Lettuce Tomato Salad

Preparation Time: 10 minutes / Cooking Time: 20 minutes
Serves: 2

Ingredients

1 cup couscous
2 cup water
1 pinch salt
1 tbsp olive oil

Salad
½ cup lettuce, roughly diced
1 yellow jalapeno, diced
2 baby cucumbers, diced
2 tomatoes, diced

Dressing
2 tbsp lime juice
½ tsp cayenne pepper
Salt and pepper to taste
1 tbsp sesame oil
½ tsp ginger powder
1 tsp soy sauce

Garnish
1 tbsp garlic slices, toasted (optional)

Nutrition Facts

Servings:	2
Amount per serving	
Calories	484
Total Fat	14.9g
Saturated Fat	2.1g
Cholesterol	0mg
Sodium	251mg
Total Carbohydrate	75g
Dietary Fiber	6.8g
Total Sugars	4.6g
Protein	12.9g

Instructions

- In saucepan, heat the olive oil over medium heat.
- Add the couscous and toss for 2 minutes.
- Add the water and salt. Cover with a lid and cook until it comes to boil.
- Turn the heat to medium low and simmer for 10 minutes.
- Drain the couscous and add to a bowl.
- Fluff the couscous using a fork.
- Add the vegetables and toss well.
- Combine the dressing in a container and shake well.
- Add the dressing to the salad and serve with toasted garlic slices on top.

Total Fat 14.9g
19%

Saturated Fat 2.1g
11%

Cholesterol 0mg
0%

Sodium 251mg
11%

Total Carbohydrate 75g
27%

Dietary Fiber 6.8g
24%

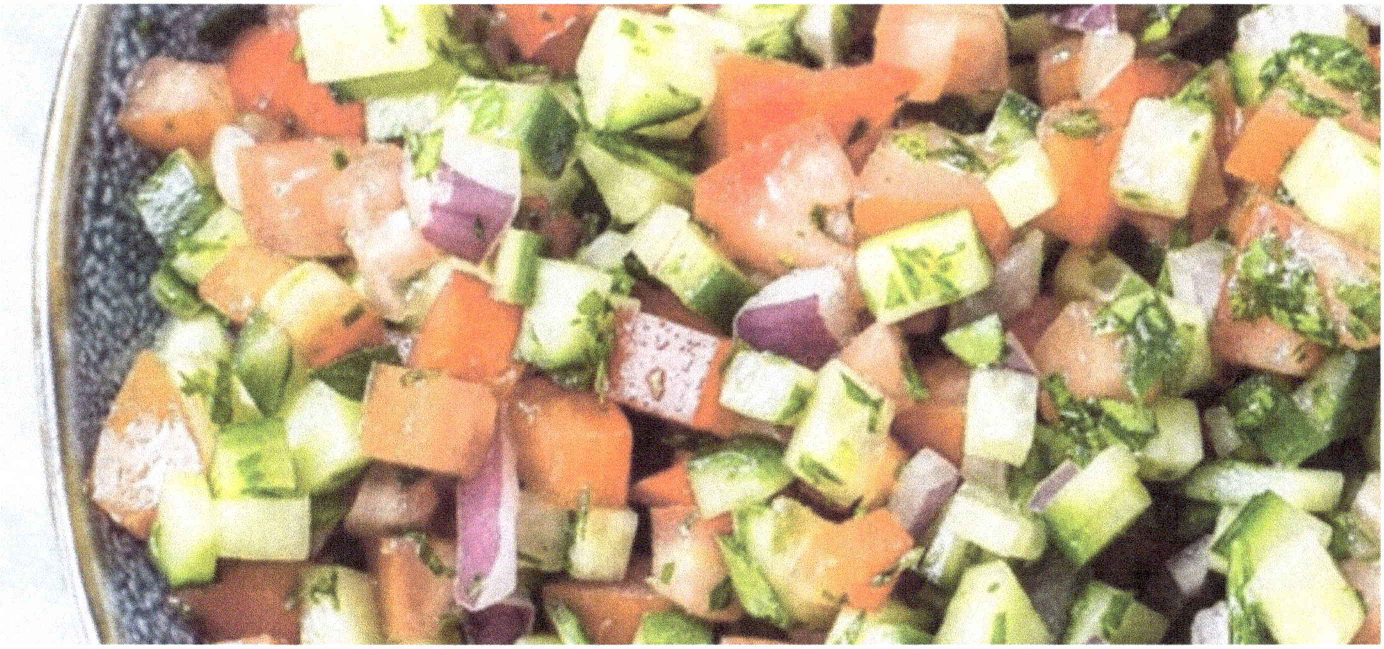

Cucumber Tomato Onion Salad

Preparation Time: 10 minutes
Serves: 4

Ingredients

2 cucumbers, chopped
2 tomatoes, chopped
1 large red onion, chopped
1 tbsp parsley, chopped
2 tbsp lime juice
Salt to taste
Cayenne pepper to taste
2 tbsp olive oil

Nutrition Facts

Servings:	2
Amount per serving	
Calories	219
Total Fat	14.7g
Saturated Fat	2.1g
Cholesterol	0mg
Sodium	94mg
Total Carbohydrate	23.1g
Dietary Fiber	4.7g
Total Sugars	11.5g
Protein	4g

Instructions

- In a container, combine the olive oil, salt, cayenne pepper, lime juice and parsley.
- Shake well and set aside for now.
- In a mixing bowl, combine the cucumber, tomatoes and red onion.
- Add the dressing and toss well. Serve.

Total Fat 14.7g

Saturated Fat 2.1g

Cholesterol 0mg

Sodium 94mg

Total Carbohydrate 23.1g

Dietary Fiber 4.7g

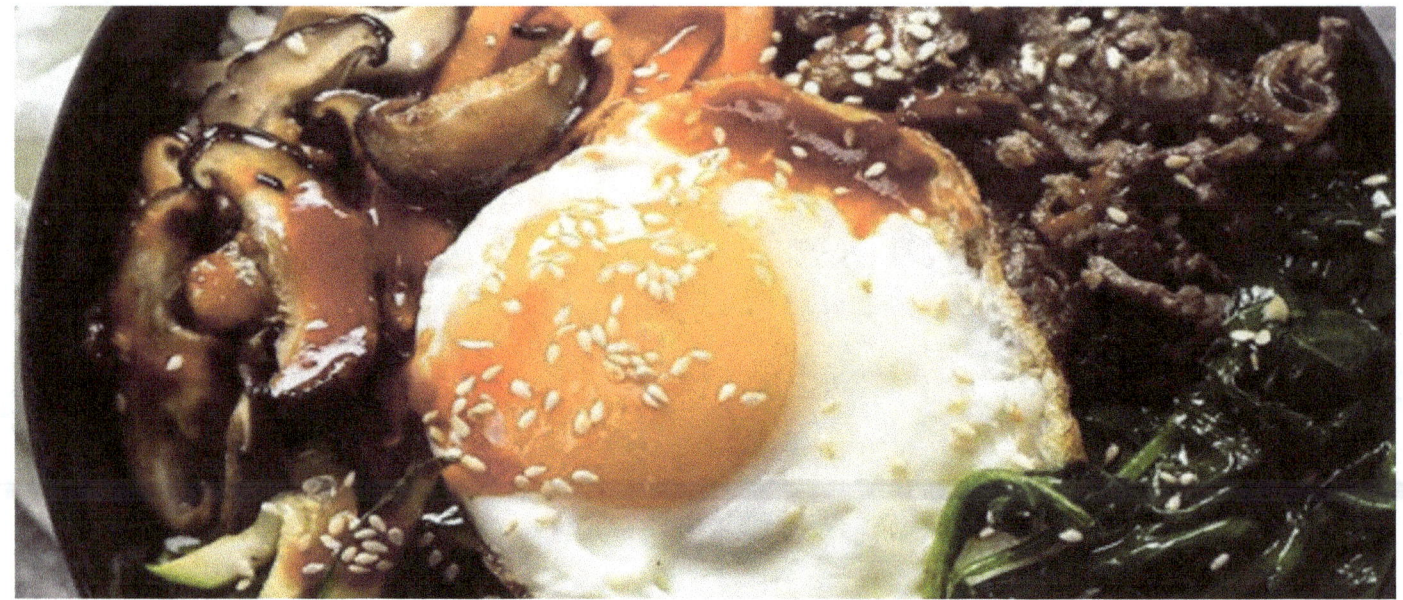

Korean Rice Bowl

Preparation Time: 10 minutes / Cooking Time: 20 minutes
Serves: 1

Ingredients

1 cup short grain rice, cooked
1 egg
4 dried shiitake mushroom, sliced
2 garlic cloves, minced
1 tsp soy sauce
¼ tsp fish sauce
2 tsp olive oil
1 cup spinach
1 zucchini, diced roughly
½ cup bean sprouts
1 carrot, julienned
1 tsp sesame seeds
½ tsp garlic powder
½ tsp honey
Salt and pepper to taste
½ tsp soy sauce
1 tsp sesame oil

Sauce
1 tsp sesame oil
¼ tsp garlic powder
1 tsp soy sauce
1 tsp sugar
1 tsp rice vinegar
1 tsp mirin
1 tbsp gochujang paste

Beef
½ beef steak, julienned
1 tsp apple puree

Nutrition Facts

Servings:	1
Amount per serving	
Calories	686
Total Fat	23.8g
Saturated Fat	4.8g
Cholesterol	202mg
Sodium	1197mg
Total Carbohydrate	91.1g
Dietary Fiber	5.8g
Total Sugars	17.8g
Protein	32.9g

Instructions

- Marinate the beef steak using the apple puree, garlic powder, honey, soy sauce, salt, pepper, and let it sit for 1 hour.
- Meanwhile, combine the sauce ingredients and whisk until the sugar dissolves.
- Prepare the vegetables by adding the olive oil on a skillet.
- Toss the carrot, with a pinch of salt for 2 minutes. Take off the heat.
- In the same skillet, add the zucchini with some salt. Stir for 2 minutes.
- Transfer to a plate.
- Soak the mushroom in warm water for 10 minutes.
- Then fry with fish sauce, soy sauce, garlic, salt, pepper for 3 minutes.
- Transfer to a plate. In the same skillet, toss the spinach for 2 minutes.
- In another pan, add the sesame oil and add the marinated beef.
- Stir for 8 minutes. Take off the heat.
- Fry an egg with a pinch of salt and pepper.
- Assemble the rice bowl with all the ingredients and serve warm.

Total Fat 23.8g

Saturated Fat 4.8g

Cholesterol 202mg

Sodium 1197mg

Total Carbohydrate 91.1g

Dietary Fiber 5.8g

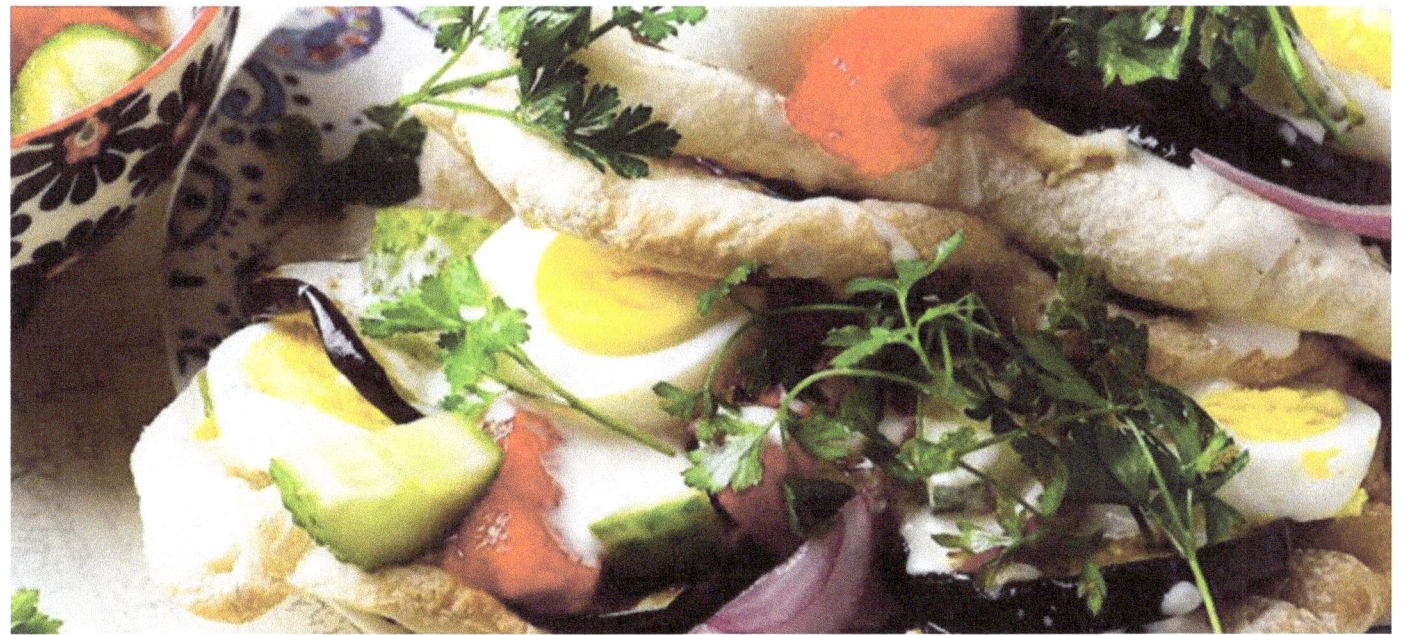

Roasted Eggplant Sabich

Preparation Time: 10 minutes / Cooking Time: 10 minutes
Serves: 4

Ingredients

4 fresh rounds pita bread
1 eggplant, sliced
2 plum tomatoes, diced
Kosher salt to taste
1 tbsp olive oil
1 cucumber, diced
2 tbsp white wine vinegar
2 tbsp lime juice
4 hardboiled eggs, diced
1 tbsp parsley, minced
3/4 cup hummus
1/2 cup tahini sauce
1 cucumber, diced
1 red onion, diced

Nutrition Facts

Servings:	4
Amount per serving	
Calories	329
Total Fat	15g
Saturated Fat	2.9g
Cholesterol	164mg
Sodium	466mg
Total Carbohydrate	38.3g
Dietary Fiber	10.8g
Total Sugars	9g
Protein	15g

Instructions

♦ Coat the eggplants slices in salt, and fry them for 3 minutes on each side with olive oil.

♦ Take off the heat and set aside for now.

♦ Combine the cucumber, tomatoes, onion, lime juice, white wine vinegar, salt and mix well.

♦ Heat up the pita bread. Cut pockets into each to stuff the eggplants.

♦ Add the eggplant slices, egg slices, tomato mixture and parsley.

♦ Add the hummus, tahini sauce, and serve.

Total Fat 15g 19%

Saturated Fat 2.9g 14%

Cholesterol 164mg 55%

Sodium 466mg 20%

Total Carbohydrate 38.3g 14%

Dietary Fiber 10.8g 39%

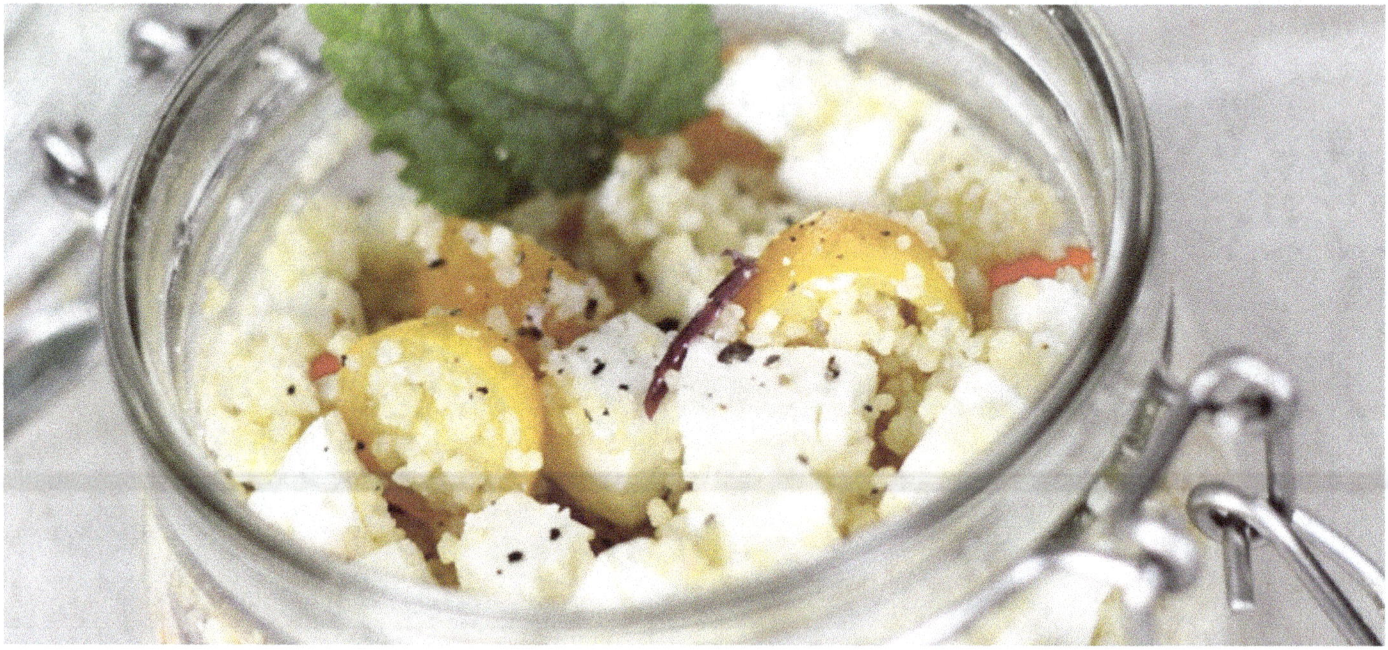

Couscous Mozzarella Cherry Tomato Salad

Preparation Time: 10 minutes / Cooking Time: 20 minutes
Serves: 2

Ingredients

1 cup couscous
1½ cup water
½ cup mozzarella cheese cubes
½ cup cherry tomatoes, halved
2 garlic cloves, minced
2 tbsp olive oil
Salt and pepper to taste
½ tsp cumin
½ tsp oregano
1 tbsp lime juice
½ tsp ginger powder

Nutrition Facts

Servings:	2
Amount per serving	
Calories	483
Total Fat	16.1g
Saturated Fat	2.9g
Cholesterol	4mg
Sodium	75mg
Total Carbohydrate	71g
Dietary Fiber	5.2g
Total Sugars	1.3g
Protein	13.8g

Instructions

♦ In a saucepan, add the olive oil and fry the garlic until golden brown.

♦ Add the couscous and fry for 3 minutes.

♦ Add the water and stir well. Add the salt, and cook for 5 minutes on high heat.

♦ Simmer for another 10 minutes.

♦ Add to a bowl. Add the cherry tomatoes, mozzarella cubes and mix well.

♦ Combine the oregano, salt, pepper, cumin, ginger powder, lime juice in a container, and shake well.

♦ Add to the couscous and toss again. Serve.

Total Fat 16.1g

Saturated Fat 2.9g

Cholesterol 4mg

Sodium 75mg

Total Carbohydrate 71g

Dietary Fiber 5.2g

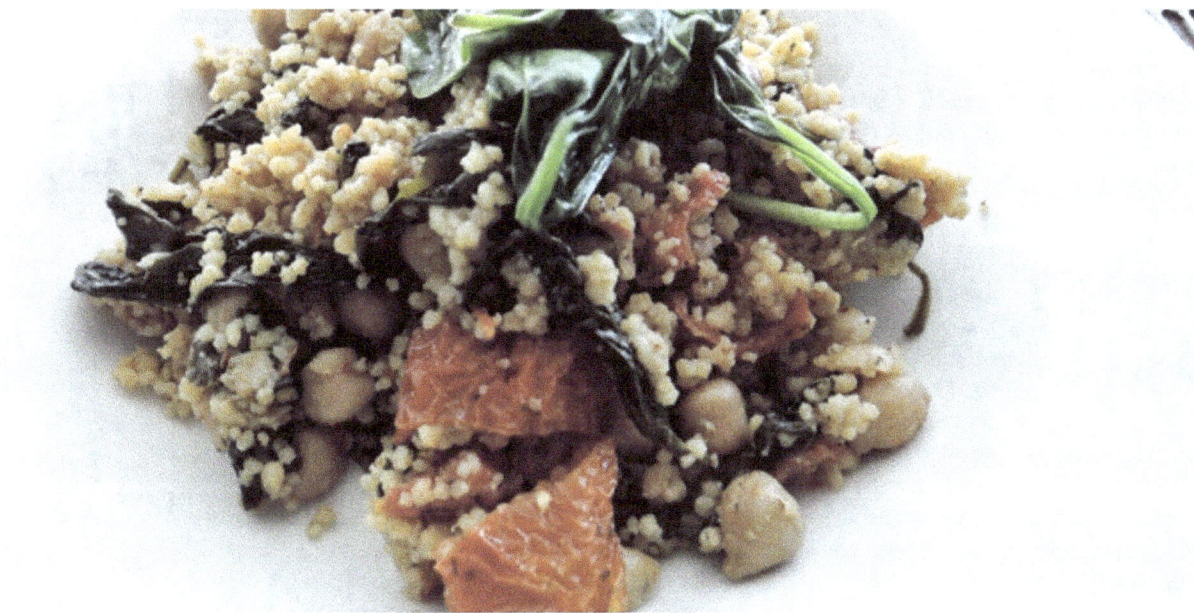

Chickpea Couscous Spinach Fry

Preparation Time: 10 minutes / Cooking Time: 15 minutes
Serves: 2

Ingredients

1 cup couscous
1½ cup water
½ cup boiled chickpeas
4 tbsp dried tomatoes
1 cup spinach
4 garlic cloves, sliced
1 shallot, chopped
2 tbsp sesame oil
Salt and pepper to taste
½ tsp ginger powder

Nutrition Facts

Servings:	2
Amount per serving	
Calories	649
Total Fat	17.4g
Saturated Fat	2.4g
Cholesterol	0mg
Sodium	55mg
Total Carbohydrate	101.9g
Dietary Fiber	13.8g
Total Sugars	6.1g
Protein	21.9g

Instructions

- In a wok, heat the sesame oil.
- Add the garlic and toss for 1 minute.
- Add the shallot, and toss for another minute.
- Add the couscous and stir continuously for 3 minutes.
- Pour in the water and cover with lid.
- Cook on high heat for 8 minutes. Simmer for 5 minutes.
- Add the dried tomatoes, chickpeas, spinach, ginger powder, salt, pepper, and cook for 5 minutes.
- Serve warm.

Total Fat 17.4g

Saturated Fat 2.4g

Cholesterol 0mg

Sodium 55mg

Total Carbohydrate 101.9g

Dietary Fiber 13.8g

Products

New in Plant-Based
If you're considering making a few swaps for plant-based or going all the way, we have the newest, most delicious options. Green means go!

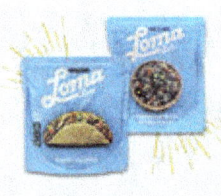

Loma Linda
When the bandwagon contains plant-powered protein, it's okay to jump on. Loma Linda has created sustainable, vegetarian-friendly foods since 1890, that's over 100 years of plant-based experience. Featuring a variety of tasty offerings, you're only minutes away from your new favorite dish.

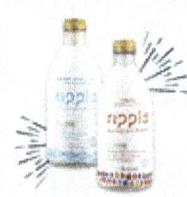

Ripple
Give peas a chance! Heart- and kidney-friendly, pea protein is quickly becoming a whey alternative. Ripple uses a special filtration technique which removes impurities, beany flavor and chalky texture. So you can enjoy a smooth, creamy glass of "milk" any time.

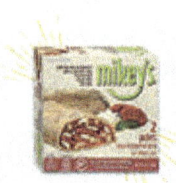

Mikey's Pizza Pockets
These savory pockets are filled with flavor and simple ingredients. Always free from dairy, gluten, soy and grain, each pocket is made with a flavorful, golden Paleo crust. Ready in just two minutes, they're good-to-go!

IWI algae based DHA, omega-3 and EPA
IWI Vegan, non-GMO and completely

sustainable, these naturally potent sources of omega-3 are made of AlmegaPL™. This unique form of algae contains a long list of powerful antioxidants and carotenoids which protect your body from harmful free radicals.

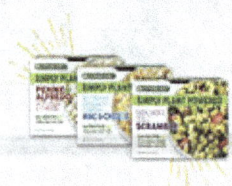

CedarLane Simply Plant Powered bowls
CedarLane Plant Powered Meals Getting more plants on your plate is simple with flavorful CedarLane meals, completely free from dairy and gluten, and packed with plant-based nutrition. Enjoy surprising options like comforting mac & Cheeze, and zippy no-egg salad.

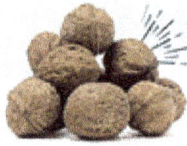

Walnuts
When you're scooping up nuts in our bulk bins, don't skimp on walnuts! Loaded with heart-healthy omega-3s and antioxidants, these wonder nuts make a nutritious snack and the perfect trail mix-in.

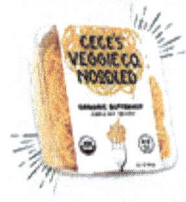

Cece's Veggie co.
Noodled organic butternut Cece's Veggie Company Press pause on traditional pasta—and sub in some heart-healthy vegetables for a fresh spin. Perfectly packed and ready-to-go, these spiralized and riced veggies cut down on the prep time, helping you create a fresh, healthy meal that you can enjoy in minutes.

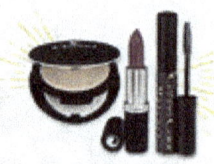

Gabriel Cosmetics
Makeup has gotten a natural makeover with innovative, sustainable ingredients and packaging. Completely vegan and free from parabens, lead, talc and phthalates, these beauty buys are cruelty-free which makes for a kinder routine.

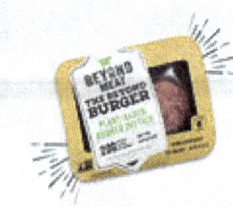

Beyond Meat
Pack a protein punch with incredible flavor and texture. Plant-based protein is a sustainable way to nourish your body and care for our natural resources. Free from soy, gluten and GMOs, these meats sizzle and satisfy like the real thing. Learn more about this trending item.

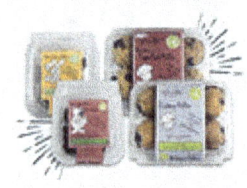

Dijas muffins and bites
Satisfy your sweet tooth with wholesome, all-vegan options. Soft and chewy, these muffins and homemade cookies are full of taste but free from butter, eggs and honey. They're a fresh, better-for-you option to start your day or end your meal.

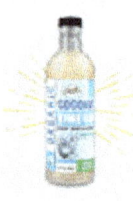

Sprouts Coconut Vinegar
Coconut vinegar contains essential amino acids which assists the metabolic process and supports detoxification throughout the body. You can use coconut vinegar as an apple cider vinegar replacement. Whisk into salad dressing, marinades or combine with warm water and lemon for a healthful tonic.

The Plant Based Cookbooks

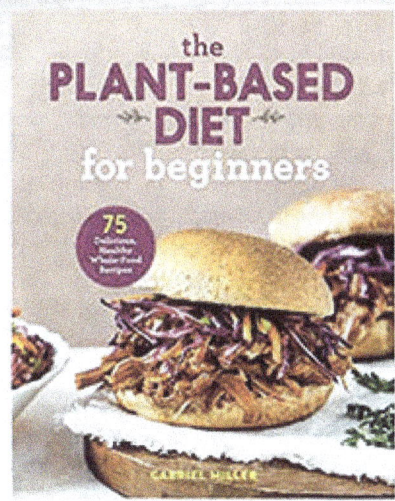

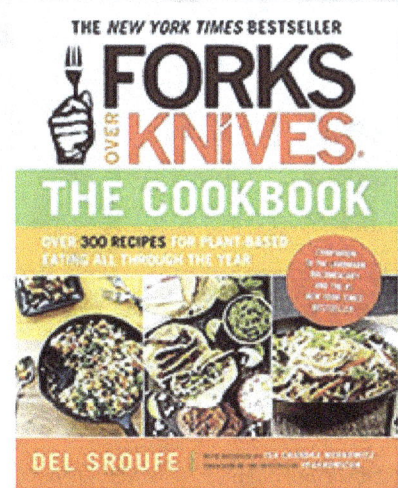

The Plant Based Diet for Beginners:

75 Delicious, Healthy Whole Food Recipes
Choosing a plant based diet is good for your health, your wallet, and the environment. The Plant-Based Diet for Beginners has dozens of tasty whole-food recipes for people who want to switch from eating meat, dairy, and eggs, to eating vegetables, whole grains, and other plant based foods.

Forks Over Knives—The Cookbook:

Over 300 Recipes for Plant-Based Eating All Through
New York Times Bestseller

A whole-foods, plant-based diet that has never been easier or tastier—learn to cook the Forks Over Knives way with more than 300 recipes for every day!

The Complete Mediterranean Cookbook:

500 Vibrant, Kitchen-Tested Recipes for Living and Eating Well Every Day
Bring the Mediterranean--from Italy and Greece, to Morocco and Egypt, to Turkey and Lebanon--into your kitchen with more than 500 fresh, flavorful recipes. This comprehensive cookbook translates the famously healthy Mediterranean diet for home cooks with a wide range of creative recipes, many fast enough to be made on a weeknight, using ingredients available at your local supermarket.

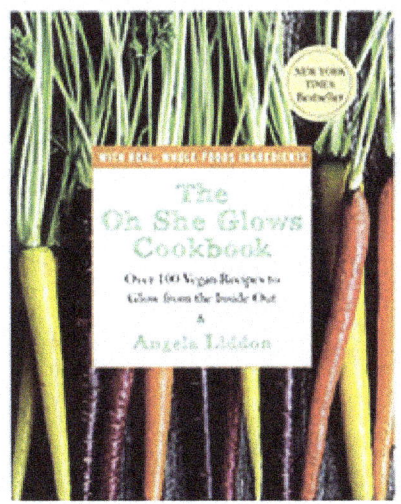

The Oh She Glows Cookbook:

Over 100 Vegan Recipes to Glow from the Inside Out
A self-trained chef and food photographer, Angela Liddon has spent years perfecting the art of plant-based cooking, creating inventive and delicious recipes that have brought her devoted fans from all over the world. After struggling with an eating disorder for a decade, Angela vowed to change her diet — and her life — once and for all. She traded the low-calorie, processed food she'd been living on for whole, nutrient-packed vegetables, fruits, nuts, whole grains, and more. The result? Her energy soared, she healed her relationship with food, and she got her glow back, both inside and out. Eager to share her realization that the food we put into our bodies has a huge impact on how we look and feel each day, Angela started a blog, ohsheglows.com, which is now an Internet sensation and one of the most popular vegan recipe blogs on the web.

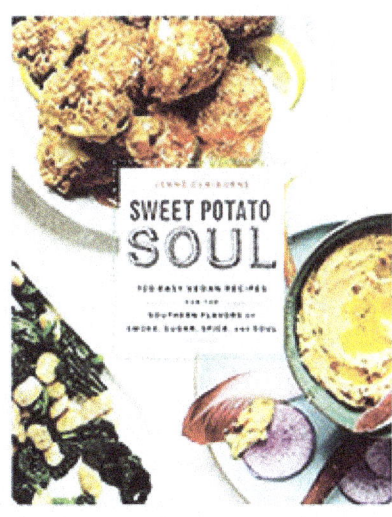

Sweet Potato Soul:

100 Easy Vegan Recipes for the Southern Flavors of Smoke, Sugar, Spice, and Soul : A Cookbook
Jenné Claiborne grew up in Atlanta eating classic Soul Food—fluffy biscuits, smoky sausage, Nana's sweet potato pie—but thought she'd have to give all that up when she went vegan. As a chef, she instead spent years tweaking and experimenting to infuse

plant-based, life-giving, glow-worthy foods with the flavor and depth that feeds the soul.

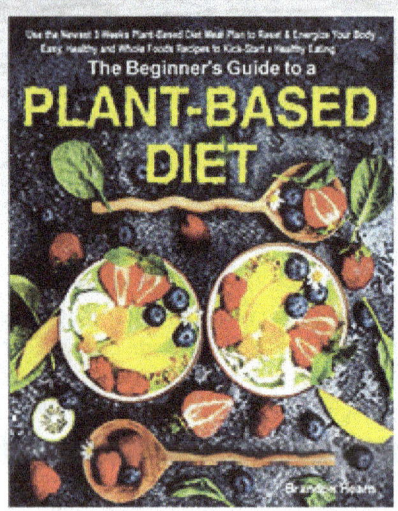

The Beginner's Guide to a Plant-based Diet:

Use the Newest 3 Weeks Plant-Based Diet Meal Plan to Reset & Energize Your Body. Easy, Healthy and Whole Foods Recipes to Kick-Start a Healthy Eating
So, you have made the big decision to take control of your health and join the whole food plant-based diet movement. Congratulations! You have just made one of the best decisions of your life!
This Plant-Based Diet Beginners Guide should help you get started. Discover the stress-free way to start a plant-based diet with easy, everyday comfort recipes.

Love Real Food

More Than 100 Feel-Good Vegetarian Favorites to Delight the Senses and Nourish the Body: A Cookbook
Learn to eat well with more than 100 approachable and delicious meatless recipes designed for everyone—vegetarians, vegans, and meat-eaters alike—with substitutions to make meals special diet–friendly (gluten-free, dairy-free, and egg-free) whenever possible.

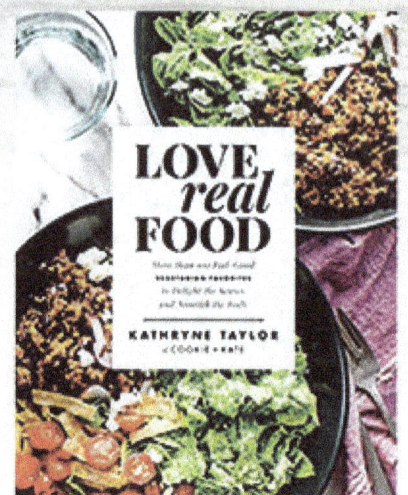

Simply Keto:

A Practical Approach to Health & Weight Loss, with 100+ Easy Low-Carb Recipes
The ketogenic diet, a low-carb, high-fat

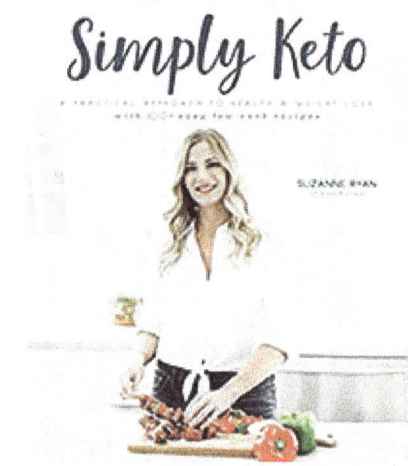

way of eating, is remarkably effective at transforming people's lives, helping them shed pounds and find relief from common health conditions. No one knows this better than Suzanne Ryan. In her quest to overcome her lifelong struggle with her weight, she stumbled upon the ketogenic diet and decided to give it a shot. In just one year, she lost more than 100 pounds and reclaimed control over her health and well-being.

The Skinnytaste Cookbook:

Light on Calories, Big on Flavor
NEW YORK TIMES BESTSELLER • Get the recipes everyone is talking about, handy nutrition facts, and 125 stunning photographs in the debut cookbook from the wildly popular blog Skinnytaste.

Gina Homolka is America's most trusted home cook when it comes to easy, flavorful recipes that are miraculously low-calorie and made from all-natural, easy-to-find ingredients.

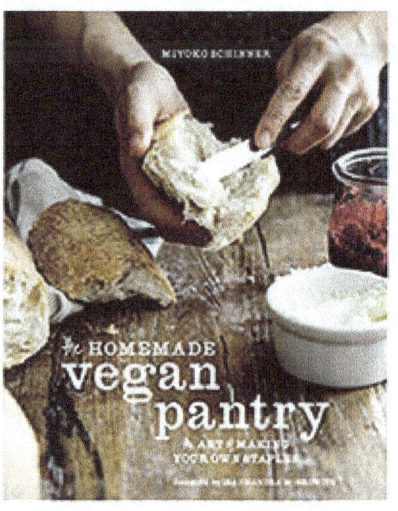

The Homemade Vegan Pantry:

The Art of Making Your Own Staples [A Cookbook]
A guide to creating vegan versions of pantry staples--from dairy and meat substitutes such as vegan yogurt, mayo, bacon, and cheese, to dressings, sauces, cookies, and more.
Kitchen crafters know the pleasure of making their own staples and specialty foods, whether it's cultured sour cream or a stellar soup stock. It's a fresher, healthier, more natural approach to eating and living. Now vegans who are sick of buying over-processed, over-packaged products can finally join the homemade revolution.

Netflix Movies

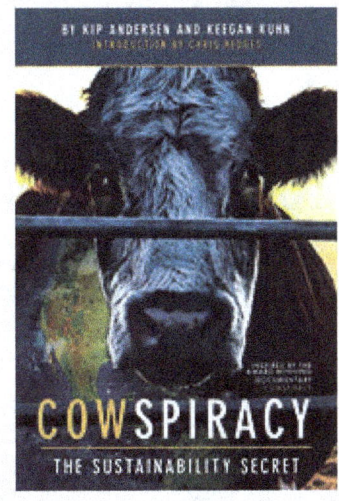

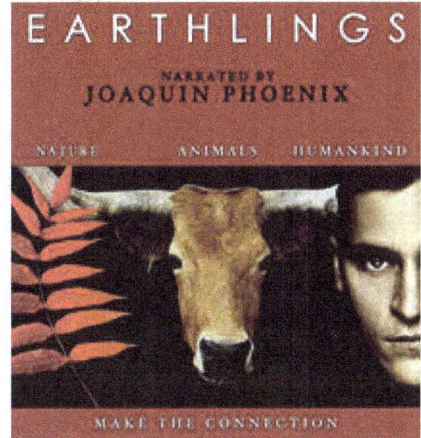

1. The Game Changers
Think you can't build muscle on a plant-based diet? Think you can't perform as an athlete at the top level eating only plant proteins?

What if I told you all protein comes from plants, and actually it is better for your health to cut out the middle man (animal): less inflammation, lower risk of heart disease, lower risk of T2D, even stronger sexual performance.

In this compelling documentary, ex UFC fighter and martial arts expert James Wilks travels the world on a quest for the truth about meat, protein, and strength.

Featuring elite athletes, special ops soldiers, and visionary scientists, Wilks unveils the power of a plant-based diet.

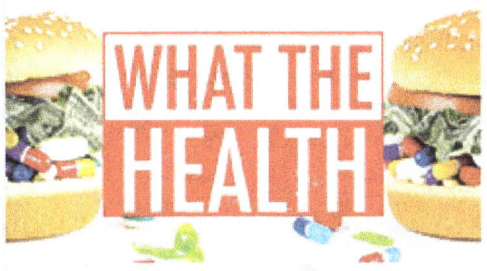

2. What The Health
Critically acclaimed as "the health film that health organizations don't want you to see", What The Health follows the journey of filmmaker Kip Andersen as he uncovers the unhealthy relationships between the state, the animal agriculture industry and big pharma.

The film examines and exposes the health consequences of meat and dairy consumption, as well as the existing efforts to cover them up.

What The Health is an investigative documentary that creates awareness of the foods responsible for a global health crisis, while at the same time making millions of dollars for those with vested interests.

3. Cowspiracy
Before What The Health was born, there was Cowspiracy.

Created by the same filmmaker duo, Kip Andersen and Keegan Kuhn, Cowspiracy: The Sustainability Secret is an environmental documentary that reveals the most destructive industry today.

As implied by the title, the industry is surprisingly not transportation nor electricity, but animal agriculture!

Animal agriculture is scientifically proven to be the leading cause of various problems our planet faces today. There's water pollution, deforestation, species extinction, and topsoil erosion; the list goes on.

Despite all these, leading environmental organizations continue to operate blindly, and this is where Cowspiracy comes in.

Follow Andersen as he attempts to talk with representatives of these environmental organizations and uncovers the real reason for the refusal to discuss the issue.

4. Earthlings
If you're an animal lover, ready your tissue before watching Earthlings.
This documentary touches on our use of animals as food, clothing, pets and entertainment, as well as for scientific purposes.

Featuring Joaquin Phoenix, this 95-minute long film peeks inside pet stores, animal shelters, puppy mills, and other similar organizations, unveiling their day-to-day practices through graphic footages.

Plant-Based Diet Books

How Not to Die
In How Not to Die, Dr. Michael Greger, the internationally-renowned nutrition expert, physician, and founder of NutritionFacts.org, examines the fifteen top causes of premature death in America--heart disease, various cancers, diabetes, Parkinson's, high blood pressure, and more--and explains how nutritional and lifestyle interventions can sometimes trump prescription pills and other pharmaceutical and surgical approaches to help prevent and reverse these diseases, freeing us to live healthier lives.

Proteinaholic: How Our Obsession with Meat Is Killing Us and What We Can Do About It
An acclaimed surgeon specializing in weight loss delivers a paradigm-shifting examination of the diet and health industry's focus on protein, explaining why it is detrimental to our health, and can prevent us from losing weight.

The Cheese Trap: How Breaking a Surprising Addiction Will Help You Lose Weight, Gain Energy, and Get Healthy
New York Times bestselling author Dr. Neal Barnard reveals the shocking truth about cheese-the dangerous addiction that is harming your health-and presents a radical program to lose weight and feel great.

Dr. Neal Barnard's Program for Reversing Diabetes
The New York Times bestselling author of Eat to Live and Super Immunity and one of the country's leading experts on preventive medicine offers a scientifically proven, practical program to prevent and reverse diabetes—without drugs.

The China Study
The science is clear. The results are unmistakable. You can dramatically reduce your risk of cancer, heart disease, and diabetes just by changing your diet.

Whole: Re-Thinking the Science of Nutrition
What happens when you eat an apple? The answer is vastly more complex than you imagine. Every apple contains thousands of antioxidants whose names, beyond a few like vitamin C, are unfamiliar to us, and each of these powerful chemicals has the potential to play an important role in supporting our health. They impact thousands upon thousands of metabolic reactions inside the human body. But calculating the specific influence of each of these chemicals isn't nearly sufficient to explain the effect of the apple as a whole. Because almost every chemical can affect every other chemical, there is an almost infinite number of possible biological consequences.

Eat to Live: The Amazing Nutrient-Rich Program for Fast and Sustained Weight Loss
The Eat To Live 2011 revised edition includes updated scientific research supporting Dr. Fuhrman's revolutionary six-week plan and a brand new chapter highlighting Dr. Fuhrman's discovery of toxic hunger and the role of food addiction in weight issues. This new chapter provides novel and important insights into weight gain. It explains how and why eating the wrong foods causes toxic hunger and the desire to over consume calories; whereas a diet of high micronutrient quality causes true hunger which decreases the sensations leading to food cravings and overeating behaviors. It instructs readers on how to leave behind the discomfort of toxic hunger, cravings, and addictions to unhealthy foods.

Prevent and Reverse Heart Disease
The New York Times bestselling guide to the lifesaving diet that can both prevent and help reverse the effects of heart disease

Based on the groundbreaking results of his twenty-year nutritional study, Prevent and Reverse Heart Disease by Dr. Caldwell Esselstyn illustrates that a plant-based, oil-free diet can not only prevent the progression of heart disease but can also reverse its effects. Dr. Esselstyn is an internationally known surgeon, researcher and former clinician at the Cleveland Clinic and a featured expert in the acclaimed documentary Forks Over Knives. Prevent and Reverse Heart Disease has helped thousands across the country, and is the book behind Bill Clinton's life-changing vegan diet.

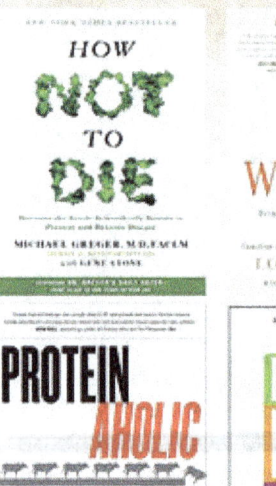
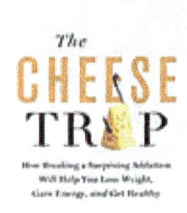
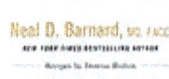
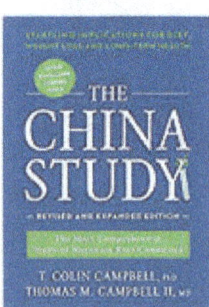
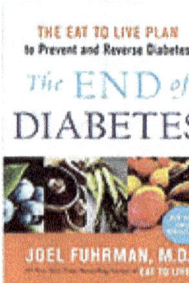

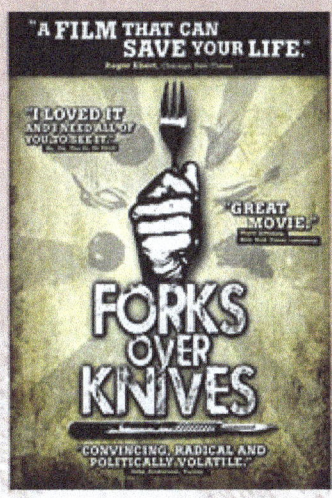

5. Forks Over Knives

Advocating the consumption of a whole-food, plant-based diet to reverse or prevent various chronic diseases, Fork Over Knives is a documentary film that stresses the effects of processed foods and oil to our body.

The whole-food, plant-based diet encourages eating whole, plant-based food, such as legumes, whole grains, and fruits.

This film examines the work of physician Caldwell Esselstyn and nutritional biochemistry professor T. Colin Campbell, stating that certain diseases, such as cancer, diabetes, and heart disease can be prevented by consuming a plant-based diet and avoiding processed and animal-based food.

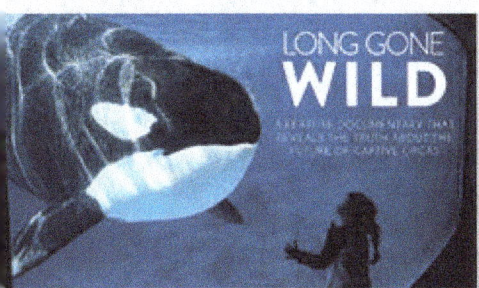

6. Blackfish

Blackfish follows the story of Tilikum, the infamous orca responsible for the death of three humans, including two orca trainers. Captured in 1983 in Iceland coast, Tilikum was held captive by SeaWorld.

The film focuses on the consequences of keeping orcas in captivity and claims that SeaWorld's statement that "the lifespan of killer whales in captive is relatively comparable to those in the wild" is false.

The documentary also features interviews with Non-human Rights Project's director of science Lori Marino, and former killer whale trainers.

Blackfish shows how being captured and separated from their species brings serious stress to the whales and causes ill health.

Footage of Tilikum's attack on the trainers is also included in the film. This documentary is not for the light-hearted, but you must watch it.

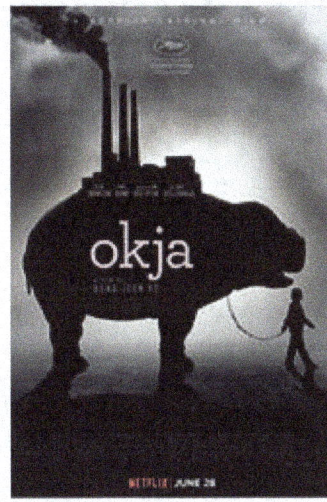

7. Okja

Okja as a film rather than a documentary, but the heart is a vegan message.

It tells the tale of Mija, a heart-warming South Korean girl, and her massive super pig friend, Okja.

A multinational business owned by a family in New York, managed by the evil CEO Lucy Mirando, takes Okja and puts her in a laboratory in New Jersey where she is violently treated and forcibly bred with another pig.

Without any plan, Mija goes on an adventure with one mission in mind: to rescue and bring Mija home to the mountains where they happily belong.

As Mija embarks on her journey, she meets various people of different backgrounds, all out to prevent her from completing her mission.

This Netflix film touches on the delicate bond between a human and an animal. It uses drama and humor to create a distinct yet clear picture of a world that addresses the animal within us all.

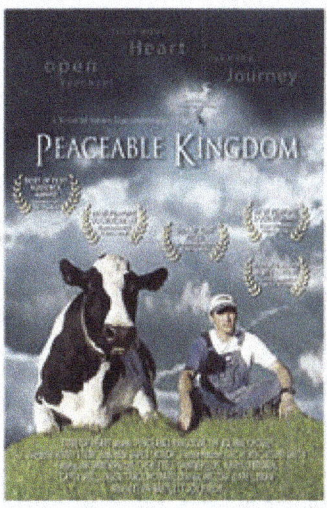

8. Peaceable Kingdom

First produced in 2004, Peaceable Kingdom is a documentary featuring several farmers who said no to killing animals and their journey towards converting to veganism.

A newer version with the title Peaceable Kingdom: The Journey Home, which premiered in 2009, explores the experiences of people with traditional farming backgrounds on their moral struggle with their way of life.

This film touches on healing and transformation, showing the relationship and connection of the farmers to the animals under their care, while at the same time offering insight into the complicated network of social and economic forces creating their inner conflict.

Aside from the farmers' stories, another striking scenario is the humane act of rescuing animals by a newly-trained police officer.

Peaceable Kingdom displays the emotional lives of animals and destroys the conventional image of farmers and farm life.

being vegan, they experience and overcome challenges as they unveil the horrible secrets of the animal agriculture and dairy industries.

Furthermore, this film demonstrates the resistance many may feel towards veganism/vegetarianism and the implications this way of life has on health and the environment.

Follow the three participants as they visit an abandoned slaughterhouse and an animal farm, and slowly lean towards their new-found lifestyle.

Americans and talks with them about food and health. In particular, he meets Phil Staples, a truck driver in Arizona who has the same condition he does. What happens is truly amazing.

This documentary is not just about health, but also holistic healing and human connection.

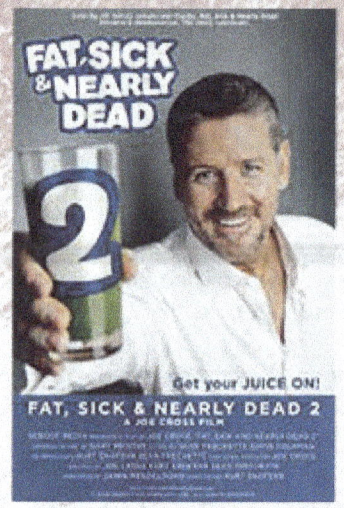

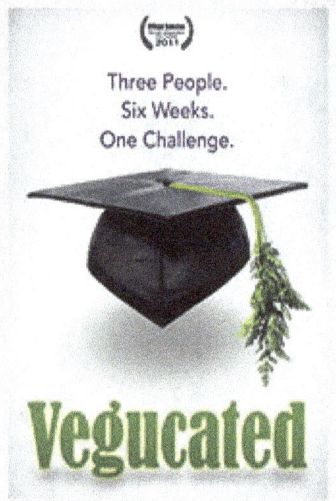

9. Vegucated
Vegucated documents the challenges of converting to veganism.

This documentary film features three New Yorkers who love meat and dairy products, without realizing that their food choices impact not just their bodies but Earth in general.

They agree to learn about and adopt a vegan diet for six weeks. In their journey toward

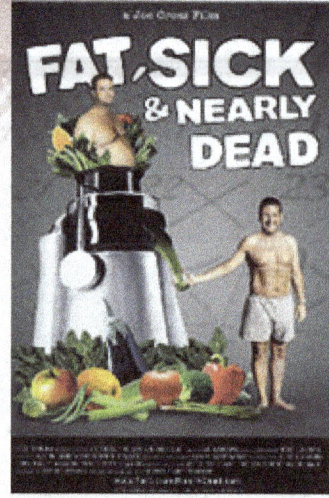

10. Fat, Sick, and Nearly Dead 1
Following the story of Joe Cross, a 100-pound overweight person suffering from an autoimmune disease, this inspiring documentary film talks about finding the answer to being and staying healthy: your own self.

Joe, being overweight and sick, had gone to doctors and tried unconventional medicine to find health, only to be disappointed.

He realized that the only option left was to rely on the body's ability to heal. So he traded junk foods and started to consume juice from fresh fruits and vegetables. Along the way of he meets hundreds of

11. Fat, Sick, and Nearly Dead 2
Fat, Sick, and Nearly Dead 2 is obviously a sequel to the first film and still follows the journey of Joe Cross, as he juggles the ups and downs to weight management and becoming and staying healthy in this unhealthy world.

Joe follows up on individuals from the first film and meets new people too, each one teaching him a new lesson. He soon learns that healthy eating is just one aspect of healthy living.

Joe also catches up with Phil Staples, the truck driver from the first film.

With Phil's personal journey towards health, Joe realizes how significant the impact of community is in shaping the health of a person.

This film demonstrates that even if we think

Podcasts
Plant-Based Knowledge

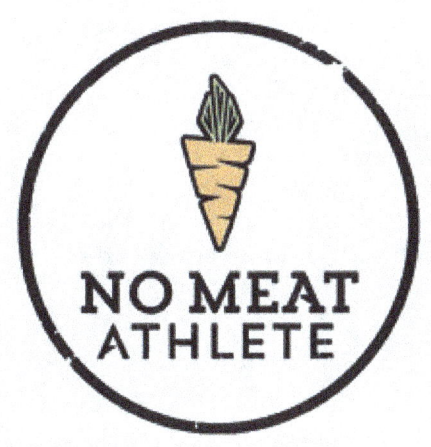

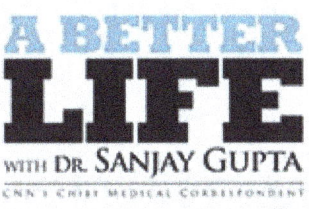

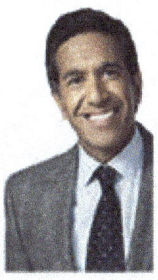

No Meat Athlete Radio – Spotify & Apple Podcasts
As an author and avid marathon runner, Matt Frazier's podcast hosted with Ben Benulis is an in-depth, personal take on veganism and a whole food plant-based diet. It's filled with interviews with athletes, doctors, chefs, and more!

With well-known guests like Rich Roll, Brendan Brazier, Rip Esselstyn and others, Matt visits topics like what to do when you DNF an Ultra Marathon, and: "Why it took Matt 7 years to Qualify for Boston and How You Can Do It Quicker." Thank goodness!

As explained by Matt himself, "Our goal with No Meat Athlete Radio is to bring you the same type of friendly, no-preach information and inspiration for vegetarian and vegan athletes in a format that you can bring along to listen to."

A Better Life with Dr. Sanjay Gupta – Apple Podcasts
Dr. Sanjay Gupta is an extraordinary science reporter, a neurosurgeon by training, and CNN's Chief Medical Correspondent. When he speaks, America listens. In fact, we wish he were our own personal doctor.

From covering the link between flu and heart attacks to the link between perfectionism and depression, we can't recommend this podcast highly enough. While not strictly vegan, he is an advocate for eating more plants, but he discusses the health benefits of honey (not on most vegans' list of things they would eat). Still, give this podcast a chance, since you're sure to learn something new from Dr. Gupta every time you listen.

Live Planted – Spotify & Apple Podcasts
Who says living a plant-based life has to be difficult? This relaxed, conversational vegan podcast is kind of like talking to your best friend, who just happens to know everything about being plant-based. From living with zero waste to being more mindful, the host, Alyssa, claims that "There is no right way to live this lifestyle, so there are different perspectives and guests each week." Alyssa, the show's host, is a Midwestern girl who felt the need to help others live a plant-based life in the easiest way possible.

If you're passionate about environmentalism and cruelty-free practices, Alyssa shows you how to follow those morals while making practical decisions. It doesn't have to be hard, and her entire approach is to help you feel less stressed. We love the topic: "How to Lighten Your Mental Load."

The show goes into health, wellness, activism, environmentalism, cruelty-free practices, sustainability, animal rights, and how to make it all work while living a 'regular' life. if you know anyone who wants to make the switch to veganism, Alyssa is there to help real people make it work.

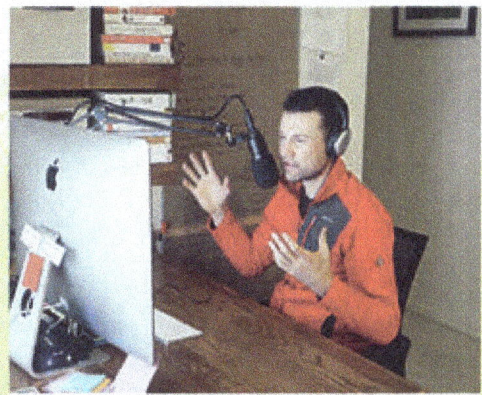

The Ian Cramer Podcast – Spotify & Apple
Ian Cramer's plant-based journey started in grad school when he was given the movie Forks Over Knives. Ever since then, he has been known as the "Plant-Based Cyclist,"

it's impossible, we have the control over our health and therefore have the power to change it.

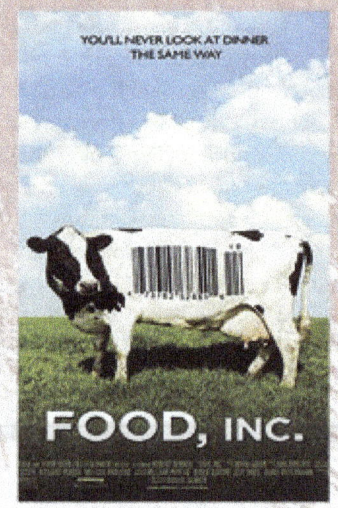

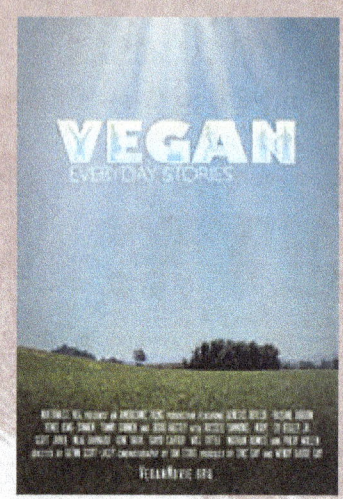

12. Food Inc.
Food Inc. is a documentary film that investigates the industries that produce meat and vegetables in the US, highlighting the environmental and human cost of their unethical practices.

The film bravely criticizes the various industrial food producers and manufacturers, leaving no stone unturned.

The film is divided into three segments, with the first and second segments dedicated to the production of meat, grains and vegetables, respectively.

And the final segment reveals the economic and legal power of the leading food companies, the excessive use of chemicals in production, and the promotion of destructive food consumption habits to the public.

13. Vegan Everyday Stories
Okay, so this one is not on Netflix, but is free to watch and really interesting, so I wanted to include this one in the list. Following the lives of four individuals from very different backgrounds, but who share one thing – a vegan diet, this spectacular documentary follows the personal journeys of ordinary people, each walking on their own path while following a vegan lifestyle.

The participants include an ultra-marathon runner, the wife of a cattle rancher, a food truck owner and an 8-year old vegan girl.

This touching film is sure to poke your emotions, so be prepared to sniff while watching.

Go here to visit the website and watch the documentary.

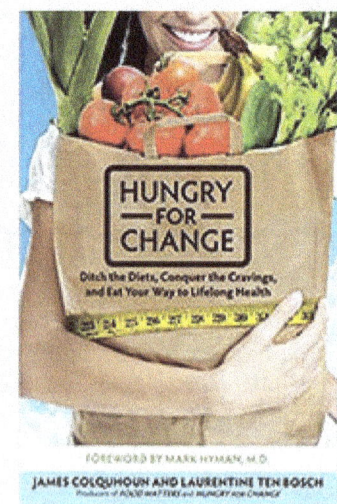

14. Hungry For Change
Initially released in 2012, Hungry for Change is a documentary film that emphasizes detoxification as the key to losing weight. The documentary talks about the problems and challenges associated with diet, toxic foods and food addictions.
It features interviews with various experts and speakers, including Jon Gabriel who lost over 200 pounds.
He reveals his secret to weight loss: detoxifying the body and not dieting or burning calories.

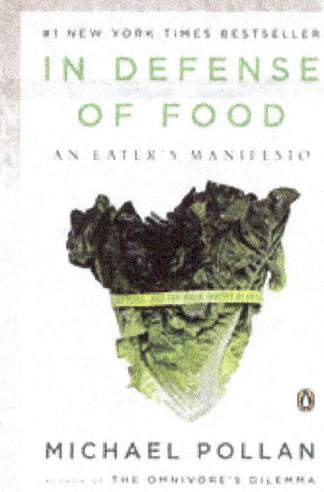

15. In Defense Of Food
Based on the best-selling book of Michael Pollan, In Defense of Food is a movie that attempts to answer the question many people around the world ask – what should I consume to be healthy?

The film explores the relationship between the Western diet and nutrition and claims that the modern diet is making people sick. Pollan advises not to focus on nutrients but on eating real food, because many foods today are just imitations. He further recommends to purchase food locally and to spend more time and money on them. Vegans should know that this documentary does not exclude advising the consumption of some meat. It is interesting all the same.

who is passionate about nutrition. His podcast has evolved with his interests and learning process. His interviews are both incredibly insightful and interesting to listen to, with interviews from plenty of plant-based practitioners, doctors, authors and scholars of lifestyle medicine.

The goal of the podcast for Cramer was to get the wheels turning and to get people thinking, as they learn about living healthier lives through diet and lifestyle modifications. He challenges some speakers whose philosophies differ with his and despite having his own strong personal philosophies, he is willing to learn more about others and bring his learning to the public. Recently he interviewed the author of the book Plant-Based on a Budget, Toni Okamoto, about the myth that it's expensive to be plant-based.

Plant Proof – Plant-Based Nutrition & Inspirational Stories – Apple & Spotify
As a qualified health expert, Simon Hill helps listeners understand the human body and how to adopt a plant-based diet. Once you take a listen, you can't help but become mesmerized by his voice and all the information he's sharing.

As I rode the subway I listened to his most recent podcast, "What does a Healthy Plant-Based Diet Look Like?" and learned so much and found it so engrossing, I nearly missed my stop. For example, Hill states that "When it comes to calorie density, it's important to understand that high-fat whole foods will provide more energy calories for any given volume than other whole foods. The fact that fat is more calorie-dense isn't something to fear but rather, something to be aware of to use to your advantage for your weight goal."

It makes perfect sense as to why we love to eat avocados in the summer when we are racing around or even training for the marathon: they provide the natural energy

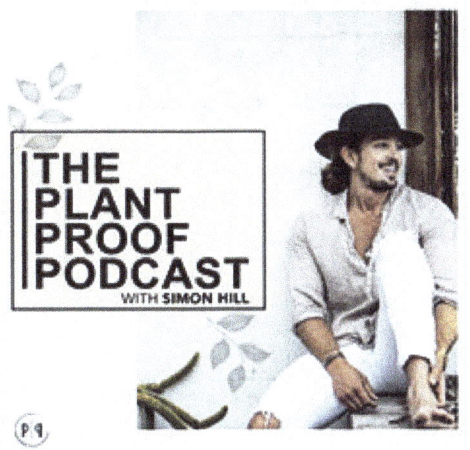

we need to feel great. Little facts like these will have you becoming a guru on nutrition while incorporating mindful and healthier choices into your day to day life as much as possible.

Nutrition Facts With Dr. Michael Greger – Spotify & Apple Podcasts
Dr. Michael Greger is the author of How to Not Die and the host of his educational podcast featuring short informational clips on all things plant-based nutrition. Being a trusted and reliable host, you can guarantee that all of the nutritional facts you need from disease prevention to pregnancy facts to information of alcohol and soy related things, will be provided to you.

As you can see, there's no shortage of

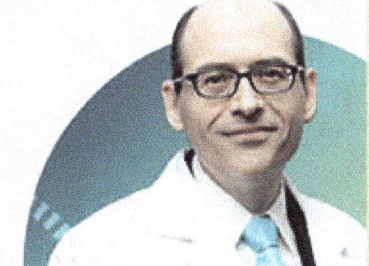

supply on plant-based podcasts. There's an abundance to choose from but these were just a few of our favorites. Make sure to give all of them a listen to gain new perspectives and inspire yourself to live a plant-based and healthy lifestyle!

YouTube

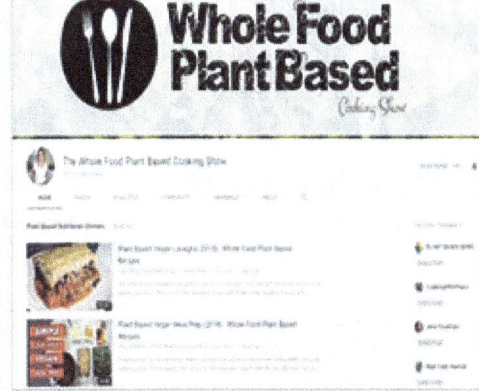

The WFPB Cooking Show
A friendly step-by-step guide to home cooking plant based vegan recipes based on the leading nutritional research.

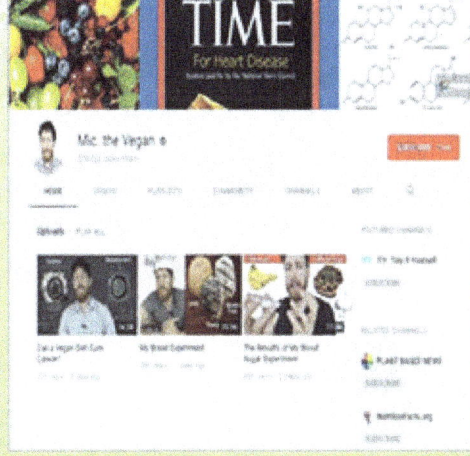

Mic the Vegan
Mic the Vegan is a vegan science writer that covers a variety of topics including the health effects of a vegan diet.

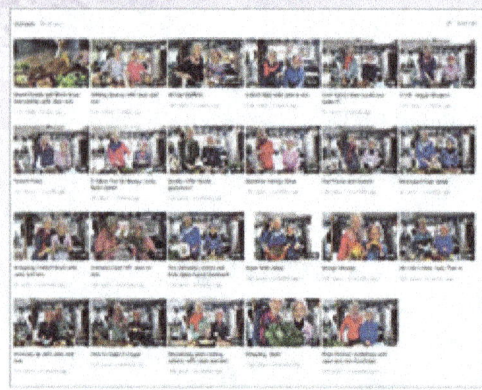

Jane/Ann Esselstyn Cooking Show
The Esselstyn family share their favorite whole food plant based recipes and cooking skills

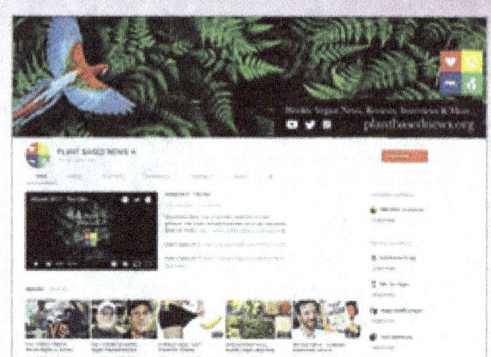

Plant Based News
The latest news, information and trends in plant based diets.

1. Lazy Cat Kitchen | Plant-based Recipes
Lazy Cat Kitchen | Plant-based RecipesParos Notio Aigaio, GreeceAbout Blog A food blog from sunny Greece with lots of simple, delicious, vibrant, colorful and easy plant-based recipes and cooking techniques from all over the world.

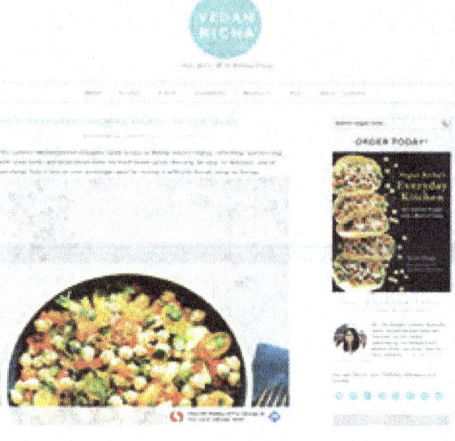

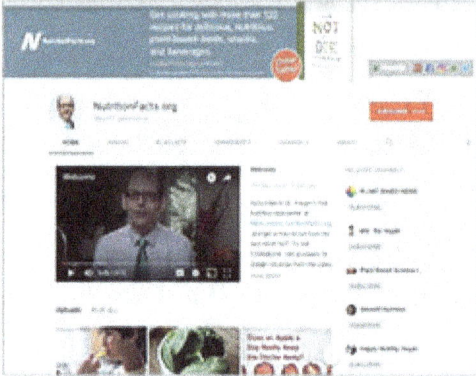

NutritionFacts.org
Evidence based nutrition information from the leading expert in nutrition Dr. Michael Gregor put into short informational videos.

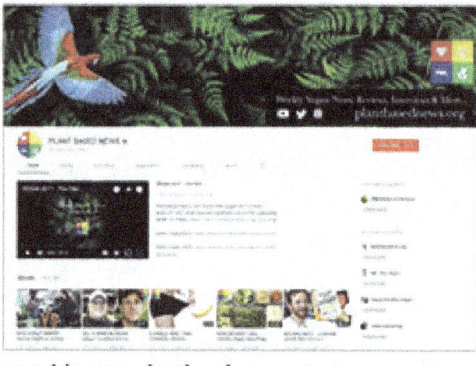

Nutrition Made Simple
What are the best protein foods? Do we require meat to get protein? Or are plant sources sufficient?

2. Vegan Richa - Vegan Food Blog with Healthy and Flavorful Vegan Recipes
Vegan Richa - Vegan Food Blog with Healthy and Flavorful Vegan RecipesSeattle Washington, United StatesAbout Blog Hi, I'm Richa! I create flavorful plant based recipes that are inspired by my Indian upbringing, including many gluten-free, soy-free, and oil-free options.

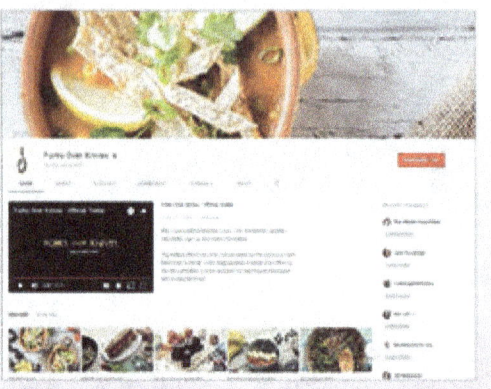

Forks Over Knives
Recipes galore on the Forks

Plant Based Food Blogs

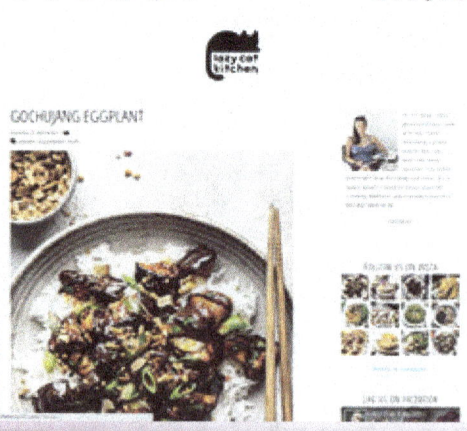

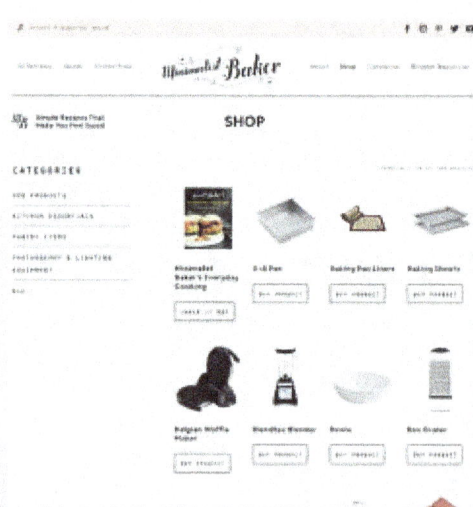

9. Pick Up Limes | Nourish the Cells & the Soul
Pick Up Limes | Nourish the Cells & the SoulNetherlandsAbout Blog Welcome all beautiful souls! Pick Up Limes offers a collection of plant-based recipes, nutrition articles and videos that will nourish the cells and the soul

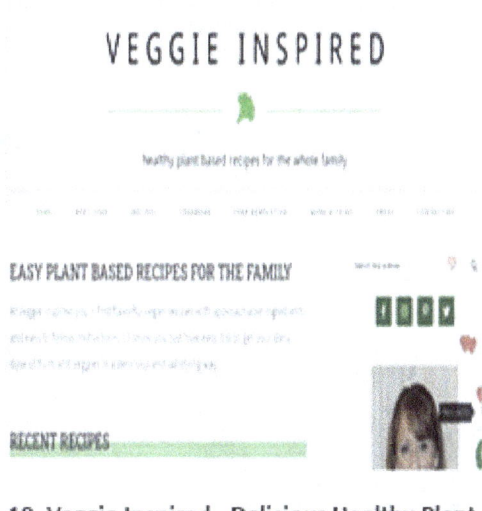

10. Veggie Inspired - Delicious Healthy Plant-Based Recipes
Veggie Inspired - Delicious Healthy Plant-Based RecipesChicago, Illinois, United StatesAbout Blog Learn how to love your veggies & how a well-rounded whole foods plant-based diet can be the healthiest way you'll ever eat. Browse delicious veggie-inspired recipes that vegans, vegetarians, omnivores, & even carnivores will love!

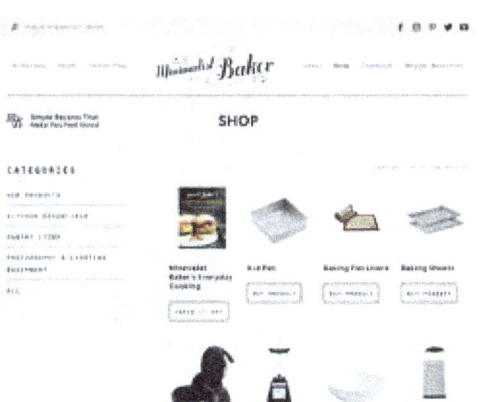

11. Minimalist Baker | Vegan Food Blog
Minimalist Baker | Vegan Food BlogOregon, United StatesAbout Blog Minimalist Baker is a food blog by Dana. It features simple plant-based recipes. Follow to keep up with simple vegan food recipes that are simply delicious.

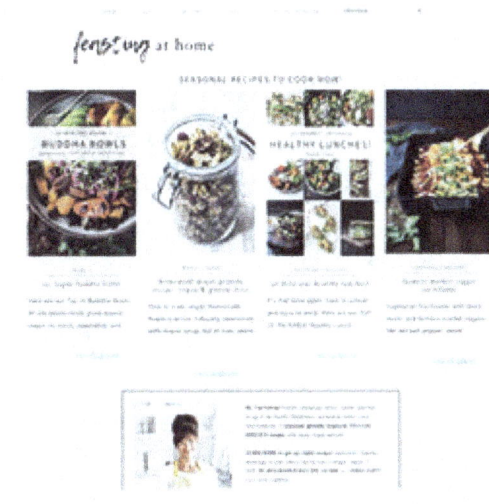

12. Feasting At Home | Where healthy meets delicious!
Feasting At Home | Where healthy meets delicious!United StatesAbout Blog A food blog with hundreds of healthy, mouthwatering & approachable recipes by chef, Sylvia Fountaine. Plant-inspired recipes to spark joy throughout the seasons!

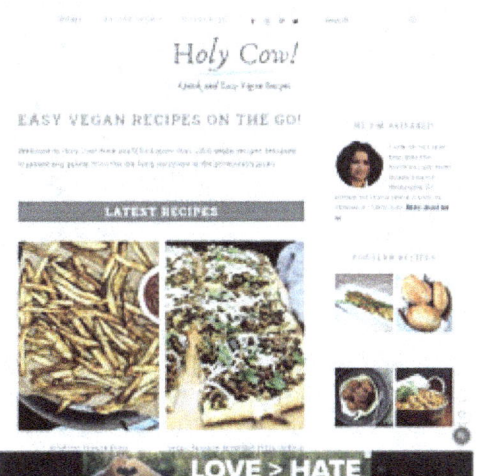

13. Holy Cow! Vegan Recipes
Holy Cow! Vegan RecipesWashington, District Of Columbia, United StatesAbout Blog Vegan food blog with 750 delicious vegetarian and vegan recipes for cooking and baking. Healthy, plant-based family meals from scratch.

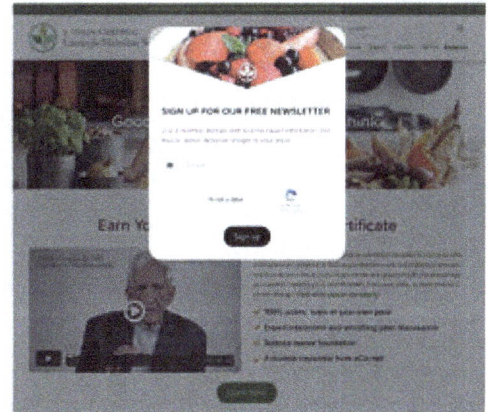

14. Center for Nutrition Studies
Center for Nutrition StudiesIthaca, New York, United StatesAbout Blog Our mission is to promote optimal nutrition through science-based education, advocacy, and research. By empowering individuals and health professionals, we aim to improve personal, public, and environmental health.

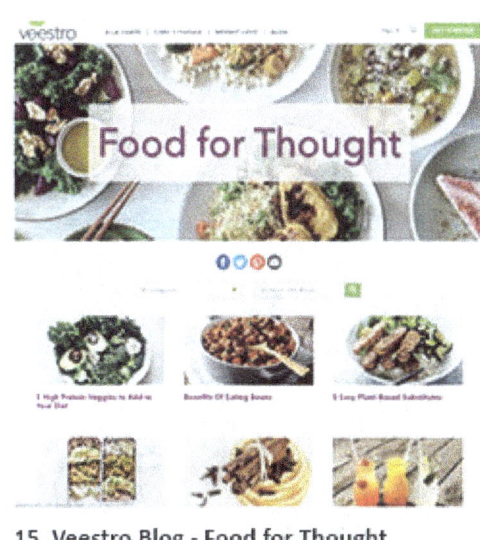

15. Veestro Blog - Food for Thought
Veestro Blog - Food for ThoughtAbout Blog

3. Minimalist Baker

Minimalist BakerPortland, Oregon, United StatesAbout Blog Minimalist Baker is all about food and it provides simple, delicious plant-based and mostly gluten-free recipes.

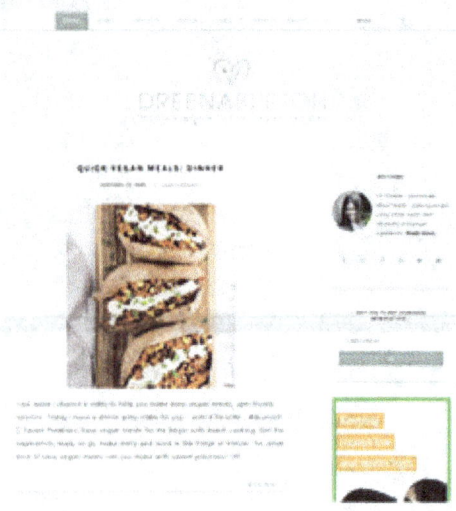

4. Dreena Burton | Trusted Whole Food Vegan Recipes

Dreena Burton | Trusted Whole Food Vegan RecipesVancouver, British Columbia, CanadaAbout Blog Let Dreena show you how to plant-power your diet! With tips and recipes for your family, including wheat, gluten, and soy-free options. Feel better, look better - eat plant-powered!

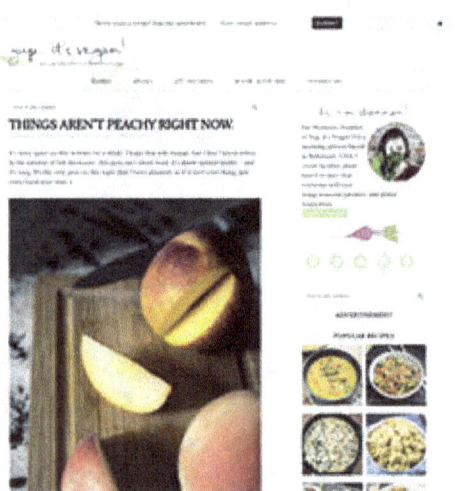

5. Yup, it's Vegan | Plant-Based & Vegetarian Recipes

Yup, it's Vegan | Plant-Based & Vegetarian RecipesBaltimore, Maryland, United StatesAbout Blog Browse hundreds of whole food, plant-based recipes that are BIG on flavor but 100% free of animal products: no meat, fish, eggs, dairy, or honey. Being Vegan never tasted so good!

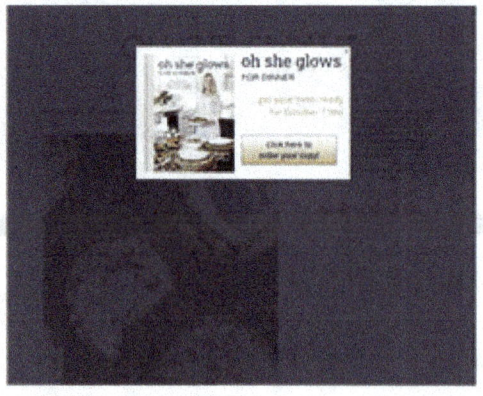

6. Oh She Glows | Vegan Recipes by Angela Liddon

Oh She Glows | Vegan Recipes by Angela LiddonOakville, Ontario, CanadaAbout Blog Hi, I'm Angela and author of the NYT Bestseller, The Oh She Glows Cookbook. Oh She Glows is an award-winning recipe blog featuring over 500 healthy recipes inspiring you to embrace more plant-based foods in your diet without feeling the least bit deprived.

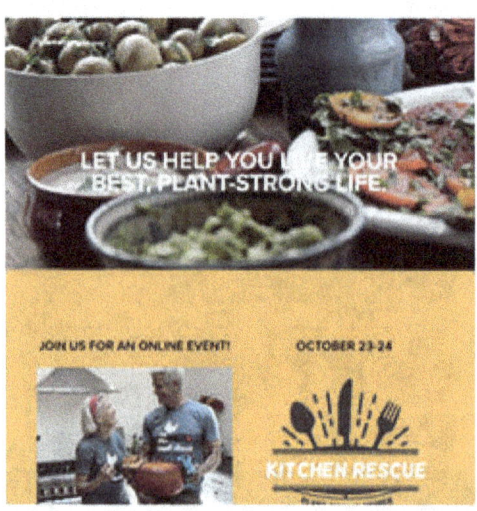

7. The Engine 2 Diet By Rip Esselstyn - Live Plant-Strong

The Engine 2 Diet By Rip Esselstyn - Live Plant-StrongAustin, Texas, United StatesAbout Blog The Engine 2 Diet has sold hundreds of thousands of copies and inspired a plant-based food revolution. Featuring endorsements from top medical experts and a food line in Whole Foods Market, Engine 2 is the most trusted name in plant-based eating. Reverse heart disease and Type 2 Diabetes by following our easy plan. Since Jun 2014 Blog plantstrong.com

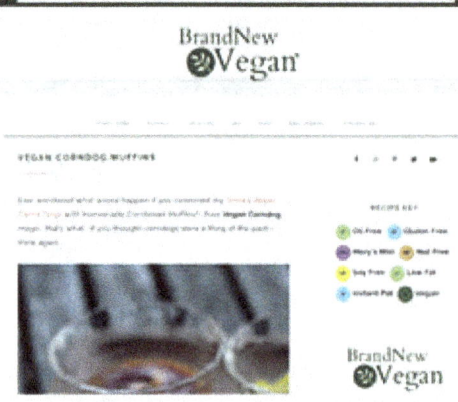

8. Brand New Vegan - Vegan Recipes You Love

Brand New Vegan - Vegan Recipes You LoveUnited StatesAbout Blog Hi I'm Chuck, and I make switching to a plant-based diet as easy as possible by recreating all of your favorite comfort foods. You're not going to believe how good it tastes and chances are, you're not gonna miss a thing!

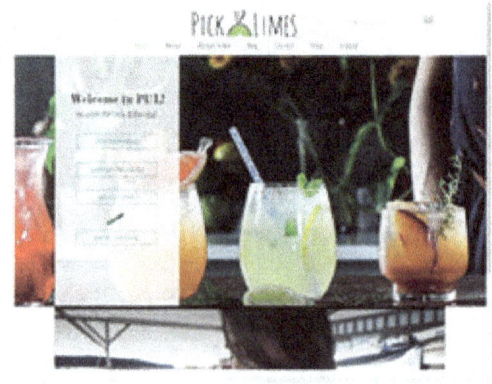

We deliver delicious chef-prepared, plant-based meals and juices to your doorstep. just heat up, dig in and love.

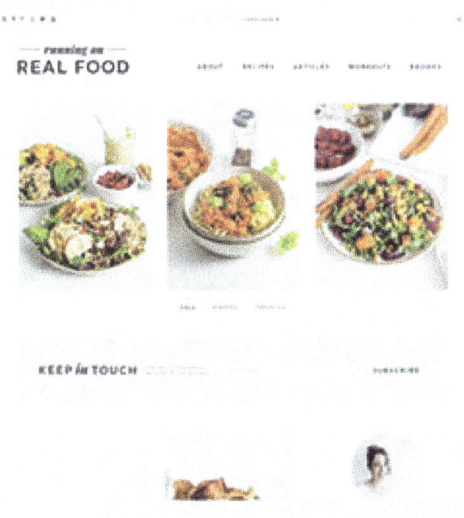

16. Running on Real Food | Eat. Live. Thrive
Running on Real Food | Eat. Live. ThriveVancouver, British Columbia, United StatesAbout Blog Welcome to Running on Real Food! Here you'll find simple, delicious and healthy, plant-based recipes and everything you need to eat, live and thrive.

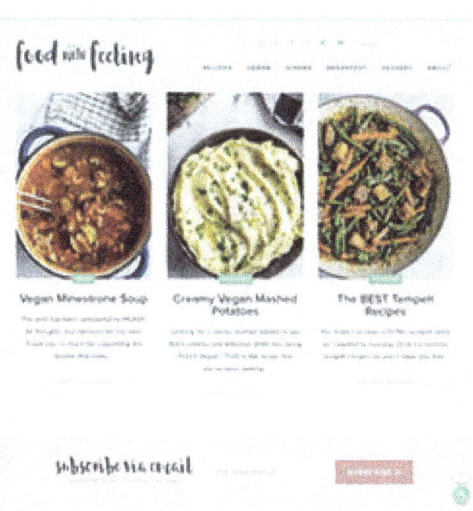

17. Food with Feeling - Healthy and Delicious Plant Based Recipe
Food with Feeling - Healthy and Delicious Plant Based RecipeNashville, Tennessee, United

StatesAbout Blog A food blog with simple and fun recipes that are mostly plant-based, vegan, healthy, and with the occasional indulgence.

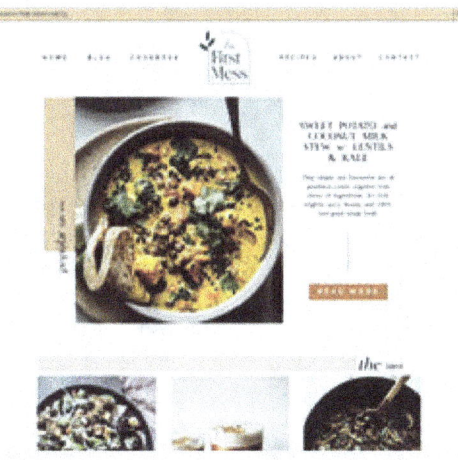

18. The First Mess | A Healthy Plant-based Recipes Blog
The First Mess | A Healthy Plant-based Recipes BlogOntario, CanadaAbout Blog My blog is about the things I love: cooking with natural, plant-based foods, eating seasonally, and sharing wholesome meals with the people in my life. The First Mess is an award-winning vegan food blog with beautiful photography and healthy, seasonal recipes.

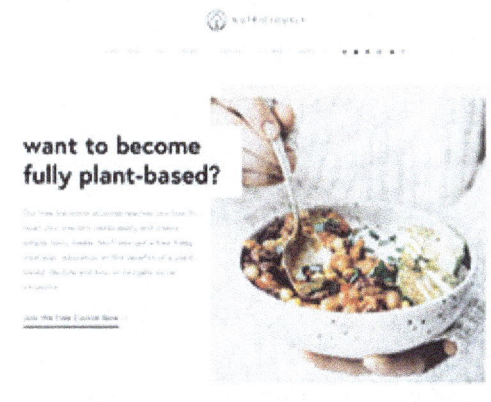

19. Nutriciously - Healthy Plant-Based Eating.
Nutriciously - Healthy Plant-Based Eating.

About Blog Learn all about nutritious, delicious whole food and its power to transform your life. Get regular posts, guidance, and free courses to ensure your success.

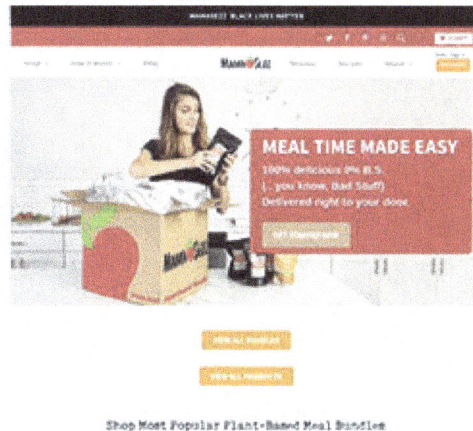

20. MamaSezz | Plant-Based Meals
MamaSezz | Plant-Based MealsBrattleboro, Vermont, United StatesAbout Blog MamaSezz is a meal delivery service for busy folks who want to eat clean, healthy foods. We take the hassle out of eating well by delivering ready-made, satisfying, and delicious plant-based meals to your door. Get hearty and delicious plant-based meals delivered to your door, ready-made and fresh

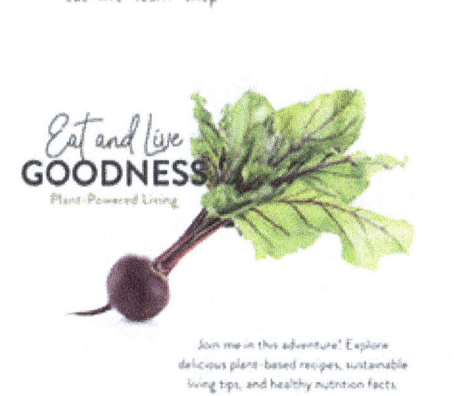

21. Sharon Palmer - The Plant-Powered Dietitian

Sharon Palmer - The Plant-Powered DietitianLos Angeles Area, CaliforniaAbout Blog Sharon is an award-winning blogger, author, registered dietitian nutritionist, and plant-based food and nutrition expert.

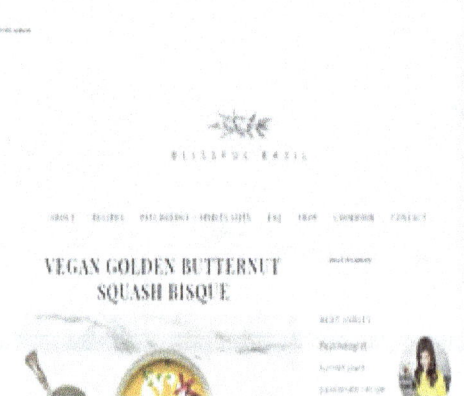

22. Blissful Basil | Healthy Plant-Based Vegan Recipes & Wellness Tips
Blissful Basil | Healthy Plant-Based Vegan Recipes & Wellness TipsChicago, Illinois, United StatesAbout Blog Browse plant-based vegan recipes and wellness tips that will unearth vibrancy, health and happiness in your daily life! Frequency 1 post / dayAlso in Chicago Food Blogs Blog blissfulbasil.com

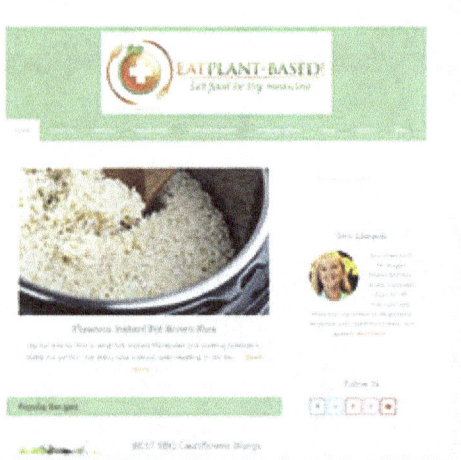

23. EatPlant-Based.com
EatPlant-Based.comNorth Carolina, United StatesAbout Blog Food for Life instructor with Physicians Committee for Responsible Medicine. Plant-Based Certification from e-Cornell, T Colin Campbell Center for Nutrition Studies. Culinary Medicine public speaker.

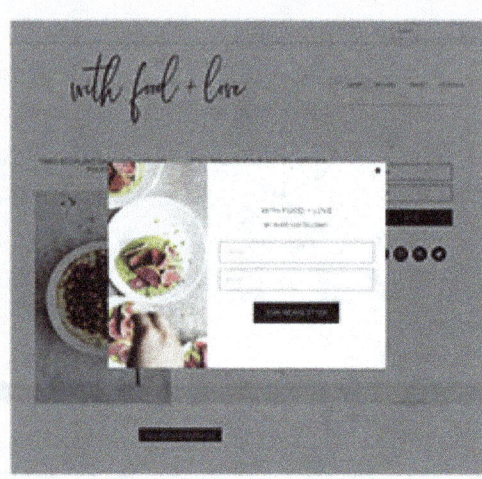

24. With Food Love | Plant-based Recipes and Travel.
With Food Love | Plant-based Recipes and Travel.Saint Louis, Missouri, United StatesAbout Blog I'm based in St. Louis. Here I create content and develop recipes for like-minded brands, work as a private chef as well as host seasonally inspired pop-up dinners and contribute to FEAST Magazine.

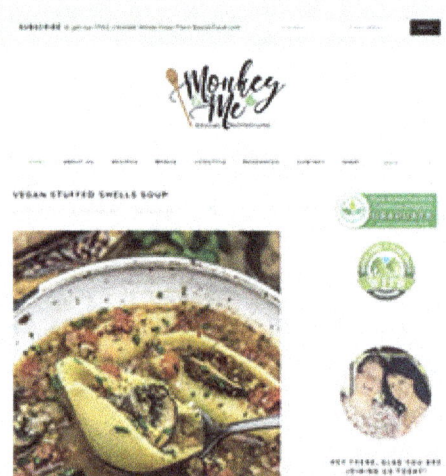

25. Monkey and Me Kitchen Adventures - Healthy Whole Food Plant Based Recipes
Monkey and Me Kitchen Adventures - Healthy Whole Food Plant Based RecipesOhio, United StatesAbout Blog Allow us to introduce ourselves, we are Ameera and Robin, a daughter-mother blogging team. We live in Ohio, and we love creating healthy Whole Food Plant Based recipes, photographing our delicious creations, and sharing our kitchen adventures with you.

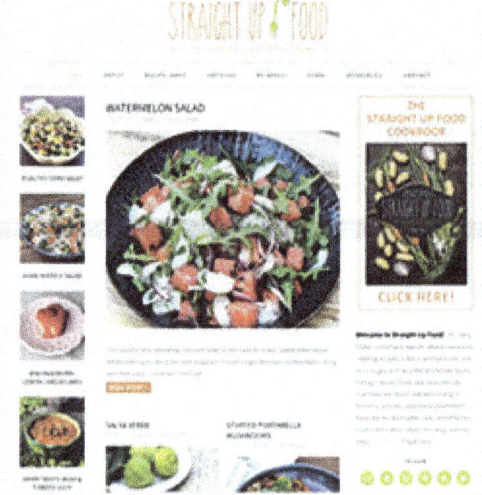

26. Straight Up Food | Healthy and delicious vegan recipes using no salt, sugar or oil
Straight Up Food | Healthy and delicious vegan recipes using no salt, sugar or oilSanta Rosa, California, United StatesAbout Blog I'm Cathy Fisher, a chef and teacher whose passion is creating recipes without animal foods, salt, oil or sugar, and very few processed foods. This blog is full of recipes and information on how to eat a plant-based diet that is free of added salt, oil and sugar. My focus is not only on consuming a vegan diet (avoiding animal foods and ingredients), but one that actually *promotes* excellent health

27. The Glowing Fridge - Plant Based Vegan Lifestyle and Recipe Blog
The Glowing Fridge - Plant Based Vegan Lifestyle and Recipe BlogChicago, Illinois, United StatesAbout Blog For yummy whole foods recipes, grocery guides, cruelty-free beauty products, plant based tips & tricks or

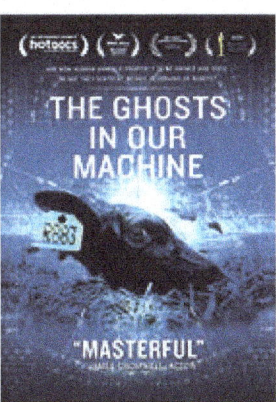

The Ghost In Our Machine
Activist and photojournalist Jo-Ann McArthur uses her camera to document the plight of abused and exploited animals and advocate for their rights as sentient beings.

Roku Channels

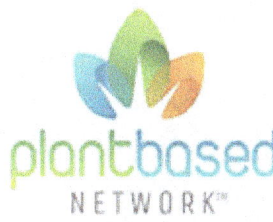

Plant Based Network
Our mission is to help spread the message about the power of a plant-based lifestyle to heal our bodies, the planet and our connection with our fellow sentient beings. Our goal is amplify the voices.

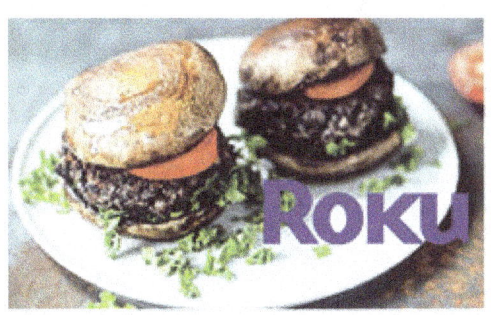

VEGAN TELEVISION NETWORK DEBUTS ON ROKU
"We were sick and tired of watching all the meat, dairy, and drug commercials, and all of the barbecue meat competitions on other TV networks," Ronnie Gandiza, co-founder of Plant-Based Network, says.
by NICOLE AXWORTHY

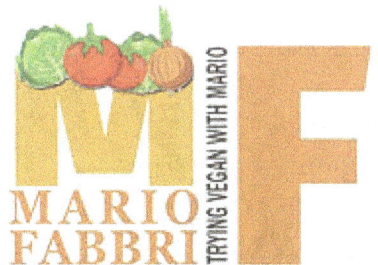

NEW PLANT-BASED COOKING SHOW 'TRYING VEGAN WITH MARIO' AIRS ON ROKU
One of the first ever vegan cooking shows to air on television. I'm on a mission to learn vegan cooking from the top vegan chefs and nutritionists of the world. My goal is to inspire people to be more aware of where their food is coming from, and eat more environmentally conscious. Trying Vegan is streaming on Roku and available on select cable networks.

????????

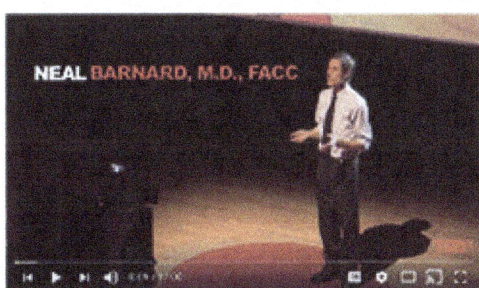

Power Foods for the Brain: Neal Barnard
POWER FOODS FOR THE BRAIN: NEAL BARNARD
Dr. Barnard has led numerous research studies investigating the effects of diet on diabetes, body weight, and chronic pain, including a groundbreaking study of dietary interventions in type 2 diabetes, funded by the National Institutes of Health. Dr. Barnard has authored over 70 scientific publications ...

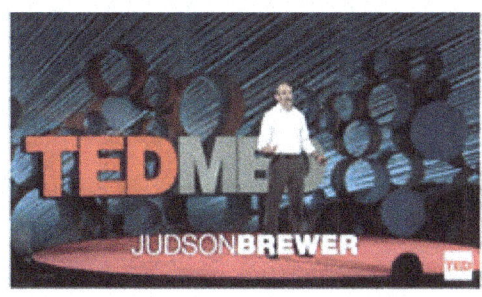

A simple way to break a bad habit: Judson Brewer
A SIMPLE WAY TO BREAK A BAD HABIT: JUDSON BREWER
Can we break bad habits by being more curious about them? Psychiatrist Judson Brewer studies the relationship between mindfulness and addiction — from smoking to overeating to all those other things we do even though we know they're bad for us. Learn more about the ...

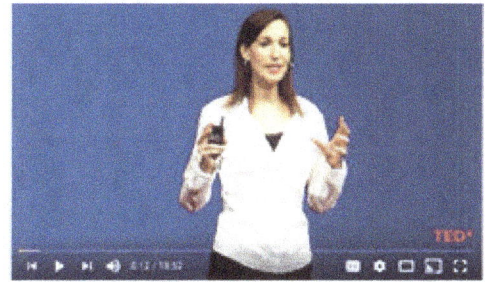

Toward Rational, Authentic Food Choices: Melanie Joy
TOWARD RATIONAL, AUTHENTIC FOOD CHOICES: MELANIE JOY
Melanie Joy, Ph.D., Ed.M. is a Harvard-educated psychologist, professor of psychology and sociology at the University of Massachusetts, Boston, a noted speaker, and the author of "Why We Love Dogs, Eat Pigs, and Wear Cows." Melanie is a recipient of the Institute of Jainology's Ahimsa ...

Can We Eat to Starve Cancer?: William Li
CAN WE EAT TO STARVE CANCER?: WILLIAM LI
William Li presents a new way to think about treating cancer and other diseases: anti-

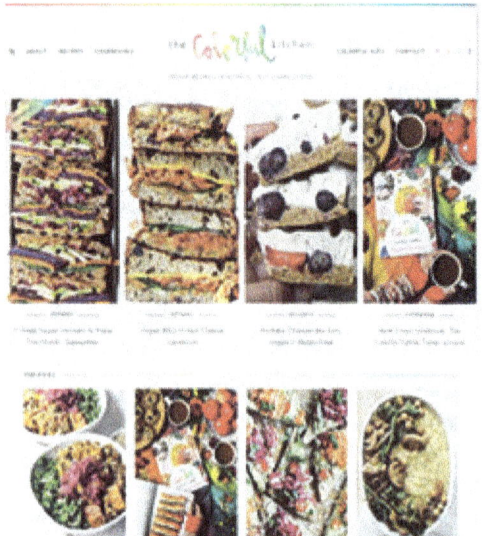

just to feel inspired, I would love for you to stop by my blog! Run by Shannon.

28. The Colorful Kitchen | Vegan & Gluten-Free Recipe Blog

The Colorful Kitchen | Vegan & Gluten-Free Recipe BlogNew York City, New York, United StatesAbout Blog I'm Ilene and I make, photograph (and eat!) all the recipes you see on the site. I'm a certified health coach, recipe developer and food photographer. I'm an NYC-based health coach here to share plant-based recipes that are colorful, not complicated.

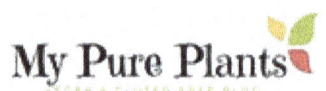

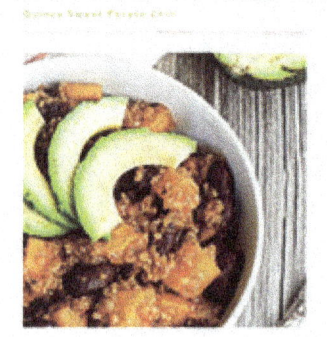

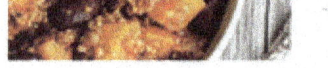

29. My Pure Plants

My Pure PlantsUnited StatesAbout Blog Plant-based recipes, vegan, vegetarian, egg-free, dairy-free. We are a wife and husband duo cooking and baking together. We will share with you week by week what we cook and bake in our kitchen for ourselves and for our 2,5-year old daughter. All recipes are plant-based recipes. They will be suitable for vegans and vegetarians and for anyone who has to eat egg-free and dairy-free. On top of these most of the recipes will be gluten-free too.

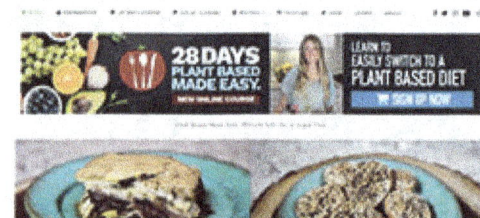

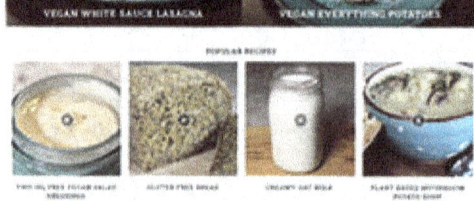

30. Whole Food Plant Based Cooking Show

The Whole Food Plant Based Cooking ShowUnited StatesAbout Blog Hi there Health Foodie Folks! Our intent is to help as many people as we can to transition to a Plant Based diet for their health and to help correct the ills of our planet that has been caused by raising animals for food. I am happy to share my knowledge of Whole Food Plant Based Vegan Nutritarian cooking and think of my family's efforts for making this show, as our service to humanity. Frequency 1 post / week Blog plantbasedcookingshow.com

Google play

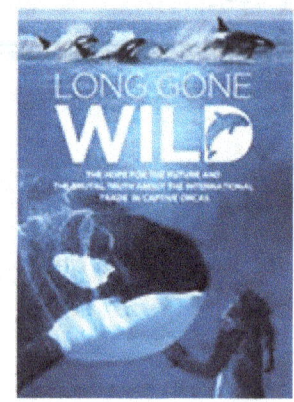

Long Gone Wild
Despite key concessions by SeaWorld, its orcas are still performing every day, and in eastern Russia the magnificent killer whale is under siege – hunted for sale into the exploding marine theme park industry in China. Witness an in-depth look at the case against captivity, the Whale Sanctuary Project, and covert missions on the high seas and in search of nine orcas held captive at a secret Chinese location.

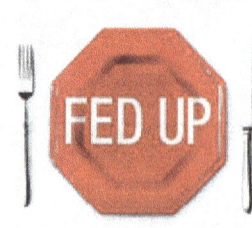

Fed Up
Filmmaker Stephanie Soechtig and journalist Katie Couric investigate how the American food industry may be responsible for more sickness than previously realized.

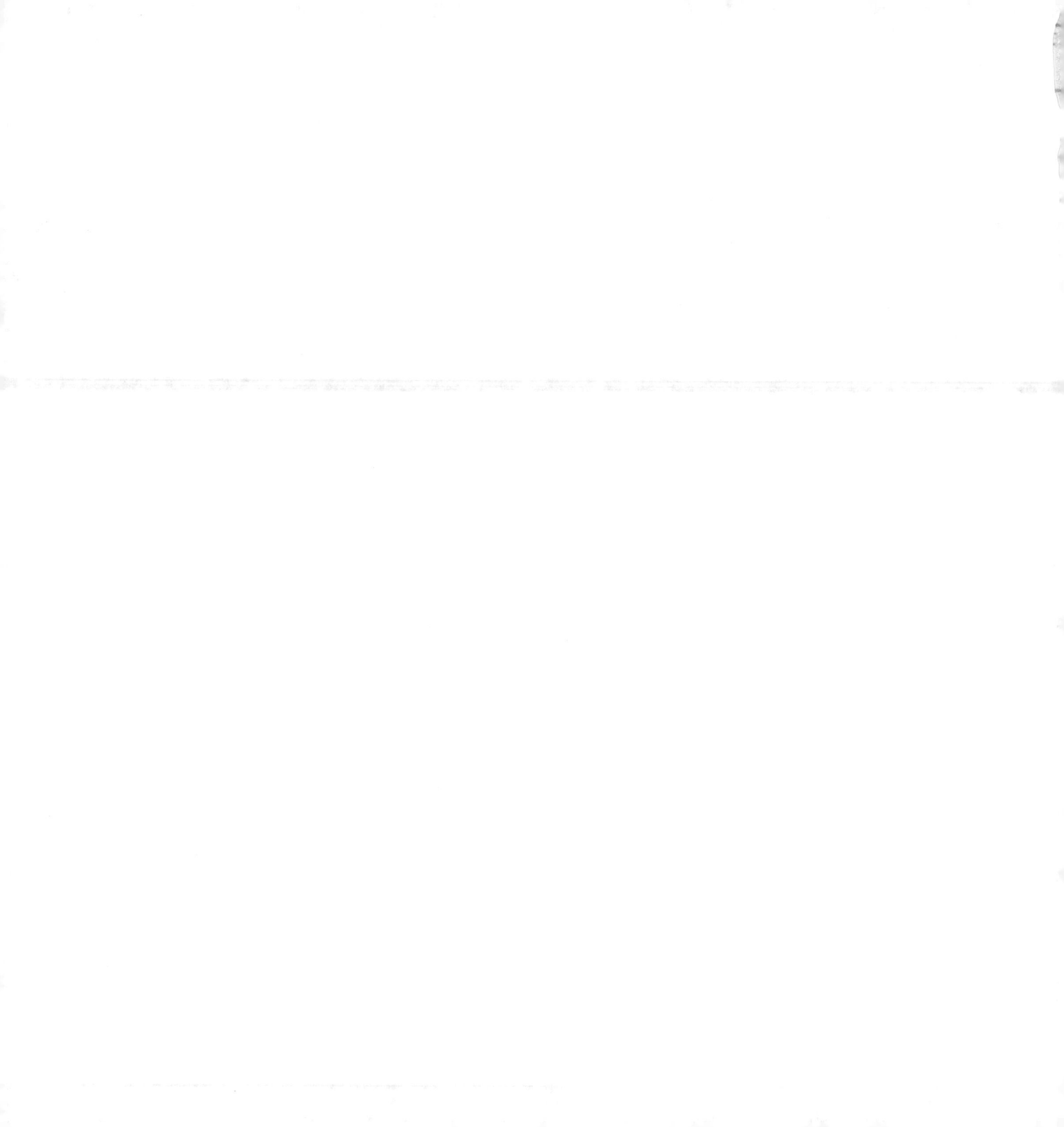

www.ingramcontent.com/pod-product-compliance
Lightning Source LLC
Chambersburg PA
CBHW081753100526
44592CB00015B/2420